The Makings of an
OLYMPIC CHAMPION

THE MAKINGS OF AN
OLYMPIC
CHAMPION

A NEW APPROACH TO WEIGHT
TRAINING AND WEIGHT LIFTING

RUSSELL WRIGHT
DOCTOR OF OSTEOPATHIC MEDICINE

Illustrated

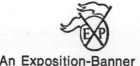

An Exposition-Banner Book

EXPOSITION PRESS   HICKSVILLE, NEW YORK

CONTENTS

Section V

DRUGS AND THE WEIGHT LIFTER

Section VI

FIRST AID

Section VII

SPEAKING FROM EXPERIENCE

Section VIII

AN INTERVIEW WITH MORRIS WEISSBROT

DEDICATION

It is a great privilege and honor for my wife, Dorothy, and me to dedicate this book to our son, Dr. Richard A. Wright, Chief of the Department of Rehabilitation Medicine, Baptist Hospital, Miami, Florida, and to the millions of boys we hope to make better physical human beings, better athletes, and better citizens, that they might create world-wide harmony and peace, through this publication.

Richard Wright's interest in youth began when he was in intermediate school, where he played football, and grew when he attended Culver Military Academy, where he excelled in foreign languages. He played on the academy's tennis team and ran cross-country. Then he was stricken with polio, and for the two years following his recovery he was at Wayne University, where he was chosen the outstanding student for academic and military achievement. He then attended the University of Michigan, graduating with a B.A. in economics. He received a B.A. in chemistry from Wayne University, and received his M.D. from the University of Miami's School of Medicine, where he aided Cubans with cardiological studies.

After his residency at the Rehabilitation Institute in New York City, he came to the clinic with us in Detroit and treated athletes, assisted in the care of the Detroit Tigers (the professional baseball team), and was cophysician for the Detroit Pistons (the professional basketball team).

Even as a child, Richard devoted a great part of his time to the clinic, doing anything from cleaning, taking care of our tropical gardens, and discussing the problems of the injured athletes with them. As time progressed he worked with the laboratory technicians on the chemical end, preparing and taking care of the solutions, and then with the x-ray technician, aiding and positioning patients and developing films. Later he helped with physical therapy, and in our gymnasium, he worked out with the injured athletes, checking on the type of exercise and seeing to it that they were done correctly. When he was at Culver, he was an aide/medical assistant, even while he was participating in sports. He was usually the one to give first aid or do the bandaging, so although in years he is yet a young physician, he has had thirty-six years of actually working in the clinic and seeing medical problems, especially those of young athletes. We hope he will continue to devote his time and give his care to young athletes not only in America but all over the world, to show America's kindness and belief in world peace.

He was always interested in "the boy who was trying to succeed," and it is hoped that his lifelong dedication to aspiring young boys and humanity will be carried out by his achievements as a fine, outstanding young physician in America. He has accomplished much in his few years in practice, and we feel highly honored. It is hoped that the work we have done in acquiring and publishing this information will be a source of encouragement to him to continue his work worldwide with the 102 nations in the International Federation of Weightlifting.

At the present time, Richard has a practice in physical medicine and rehabilitation in Miami, Florida. He is attending physician at the University School of Medicine in the department of orthopedics and rehabilitation, and is a former fellow in rehabilitation medicine at the Institute of Rehabilitation Medicine, New York University.

PREFACE

"It is better to light a candle
than to curse the darkness . . ."

The last picture in this book of the candle and the saying underneath it was given to me by my mother when I first began my practice. I placed it in my office, and there it has remained through the years. I have treasured it and try to live by it.

The lighting of the great Olympic torch from the eternal flame every four years is significant of the world's being lighted; the darkness and despair vanish and give way to a new awakening of friendship and fellowship among sportsmen and sportswomen throughout the world. These men and women live, work, play, dine, and socialize together; there are no international boundaries in the Olympic Village.

If one were to look at the world from outer space and see one spot from where all the earth's activities radiated, one might see a great, glowing funnel of triumph and energy. This funnel would be the Olympic Games. How wonderful to know that *you* can be a part of them, as a competitor, official, or onlooker. During the Olympics, millions of people the world over have a common interest; they are bound together by sports. Surely the rekindling of the Olympics every four years is the unsurpassed inspiration of mankind.

Thousands of athletes, the finest the world over, parade into the great stadium. They are led by representatives of Greece, followed by the representatives of the other nations. They march in alphabetical order, and the host nation enters last. What a sight! Flags and banners flying high . . . colorful uniforms brightening the field. The torch is lit and the birds of peace released; balloons soar high.

The host country itself puts on its Sunday best. New roads are built, and subway, bus and train service are at their peak. The Olympic Village is built for the athlete who has reached his goal—has he really made it to the Olympics?

When were the first Olympics held? Imagine Greece about 1200 B.C. Think of the great encounters over the years among the Spartans, Athenians, the men of Delphi and Crete, the Minoans. This was a time of invasion and warfare, yet, in spite of these, the Olympics lived until about A.D. 395. Then the spirit of the Olympics slept for over a thousand years and was awakened in 1896 by Baron de Coubertin. This was one of the greatest accomplishments of his century—the flame was rekindled, and the world, once again, was brought together in peace.

Goodwill, love, understanding, and harmony become bywords at the Olympics. The athlete becomes his brother's keeper. What a feeling to see athletes from different countries helping one another. I've seen one athlete apply first aid and give advice to another, and then see the recipient of the aid cry for the friend who helped him and lost.

Here is the true spirit of fellowship, and what better place to rejuvenate this feeling in self and others than the Olympics.

ACKNOWLEDGMENTS

There are so many people to whom I am very grateful for their support and help through the years. My wife, Dorothy Gay, my daughter Dorothy Gay Vela, and my granddaughter Dorothy Gay Vela III were an endless source of help and encouragement; my wife and daughter were a great assistance in the preparation of notes and with photography. Others include Honorary I.W.F. Life President Clarence Johnson; Olympic coach Bob Hoffman; General Secretary of the I.W.F. Oscar State; coach and teacher Morris Weissbrot; news commentator Dave Diles; John Terpak; Rudy Sablo; Don Graham; trainers Dick Smith and Carl Faeth; Dave Matlin; Dennis Reno; Dr. Richard You; Russ Knipp; Carl Miller; Luis Russell Vela, Jr.; Dr. Philip Greenman; Dave Mayor; Joe Falls; Vince Doyle; Hal Middlesworth; Bob Crist; Murray Levin; Frank Bates; and finally my son, Richard, to whom this book is dedicated.

Section I

WEIGHT-TRAINING EXERCISES

THE WARM-UP
AND CONDITIONING SESSION

Weight training should strengthen weak muscles, especially in areas lacking adequate flexibility. The young athlete must be ready for the tasks he is expected to perform, especially when he's expected to do better than he's ever done before. In his warm-up or conditioning session, one should exert every energy to adequately prepare his respiratory, circulatory, and neuromuscular systems for the forthcoming events in which he must participate. It is especially important to have a warm-up session before a boy enters a meet, especially if he is in an area where the room temperature might be 60° or 65°, or if he has been working out and then slows down.

Many times a boy waiting on a stool or a bench will get a cramp. Instruct this athlete to keep warm and limber, and be ready at all times. You may think you are fifth or sixth in line, and, all of a sudden, with the shifting and changing of the amount of weights, you are the next lifter; so be prepared, be warm, and have your condition at its peak.

In order to assure peak condition, here are a few suggestions which I have found to be adequate in my many years of working with athletes. I have chosen specific areas of the body and have developed exercise programs for each.

One area usually found to be weak is the shoulder, more specifically, the muscles of the shoulder controlling rotation movements. This group of muscles usually is injured by a sudden fall.

These two basic exercises have proved to be beneficial in strengthening the shoulder. For the first exercise, position the boy on his back, with his arms adducted or pulled close to form 90° angles, and his forearm also flexed to 90°. The palm is placed in front on a table, and resistance is given at the wrist as the boy attempts to roll or lift his arm up over and back. In the second exercise, the backs of the hands are placed down as the arm is rolled back up over the head; the resistance is again given at the wrist, and the athlete attempts to roll the arm up and backward (see figs. 1a, 1b, and 1c).

3

Figs. 1a, 1b, 1c. External rotation at shoulder

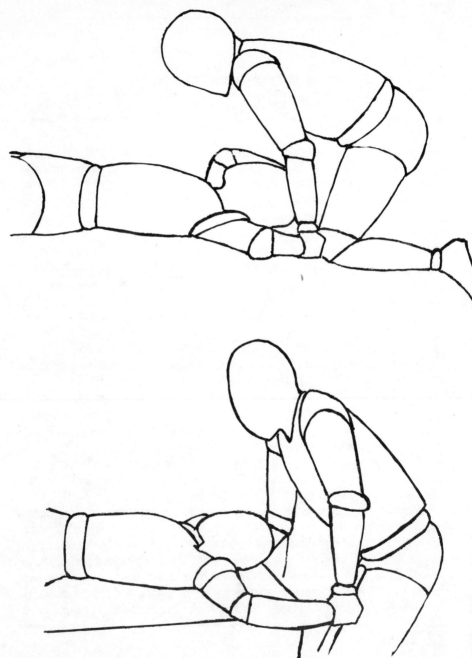

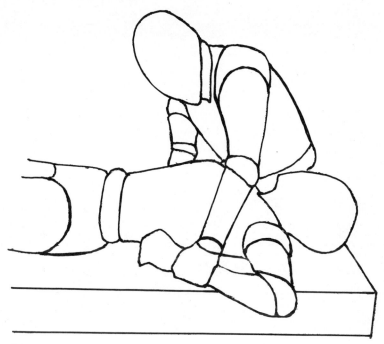

These exercises can also be done isotonically by using dumbbells for resistance. The flexibility of the rotator musculature is also very important, and I suggest that the second set of exercises be used with slightly heavier weights to stretch the rotator musculature (see fig. 2).

A strong abdominal region greatly assists hip flexion; it supports the abdominal viscera and aids in correct posture of the lumbosacral region of the spine. Thus, the abdominal musculature is vastly important. Exercises for strengthening this area are sit-ups from the hook-lying position (see fig. 3) and the knee-to-chest jump (see fig. 4).

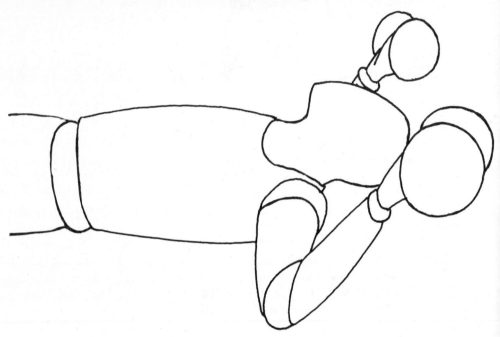

Fig. 2. Rotation with weights

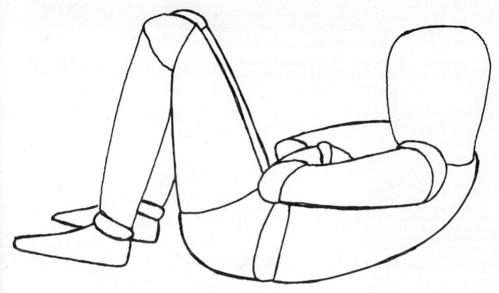

Fig. 3. Sit-up for hook-lying position

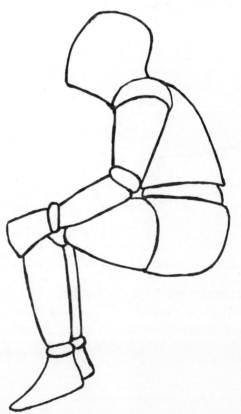

Fig. 4. Knee-to-chest jump

The forearms and the hands are vitally important to the athlete and should be given special attention. Strength in these areas cannot be minimized. One of the best static isometric exercises for the hands and the forearms is the fingertip push. A good exercise for the athlete to do on his own is the exercise which uses the wrist roller. Be sure to roll the

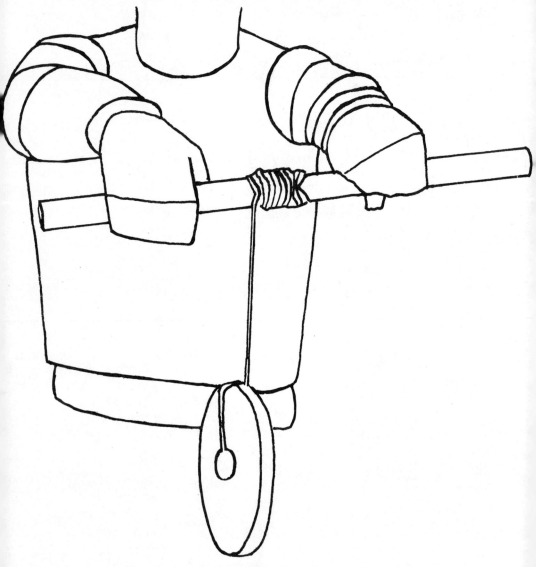

Fig. 5. Wrist roller

bar in both directions up and down, first using about two pounds, then three, four, five, and rolling the bar, holding your arms out straight in front of you, and rolling this weight from the floor, then unwinding it slowly, and rolling it back down (see fig. 5). This is an excellent exercise for the forearms and wrist.

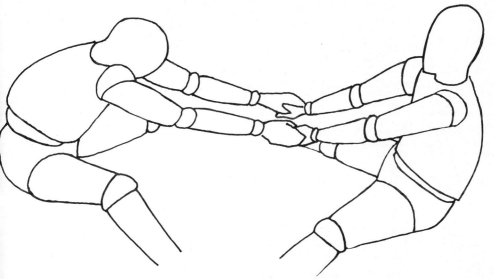

Fig. 6. Adductor test and stretch

The pushup has always been one of the finest exercises, but one thing to remember in doing this is to have the individual shift his weight to the thumb or the fingertips. Adequate strength of the hands, primarily the thumbs, should prevent many injuries to the area. A bad injury at the base of the thumb can disable an athlete for anywhere from a week to a month.

Another area where flexibility is our primary target is the groin, or adductor, of the thigh area. Many of our lifters showed inadequate strength in this area and a lack of flexibility when tested (see fig. 6).

The best exercise for stretching this area uses the same test, with an alternate force from one person to another. The boy should be able to place his forehead within 6 inches of the floor without flexing his knees or bringing his legs together.

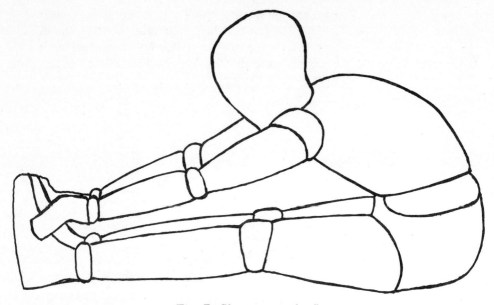

*Fig. 7. Shoes on and off
from long-sitting position*

Another area where adequate strength is usually found but flexibility is absent is in the posterior thigh or the hamstring musculature. Every exercise program should include the strengthening of these muscles. I can't think of one weight-lifting meet where I haven't treated someone for a torn or frayed hamstring. Nothing will cut down your efficiency more than a pulled hamstring.

There are two exercises for acquiring and maintaining the flexibility of this musculature. One, for lack of a better name, is called the toe-toucher, where you sit, reach out, and touch your toes. A second one, and always a good thing to do, is to untie and tie your shoes in this position. Upon arising in the morning, there is nothing better than a good stretch, and each time you tie your shoes you give the hamstring an excellent workout (see fig. 7).

The opposite area of the thigh, the front of your leg, and other muscles of the quadriceps are of vital importance to all athletes. We recognize the importance of adequate strength in these muscles for the normal performance of the lower extremities. Strength and flexibility are vitally important. A good exercise to do in an individual program is the squat. Go down ¾ of the way, extending your hands straight out in front; then place weight on your back—a bar with 25 lbs. to 50 lbs. on it —and do ¾ squats with this weight on the shoulders. One excellent exercise is running up stairs—never down—first one and then two at a

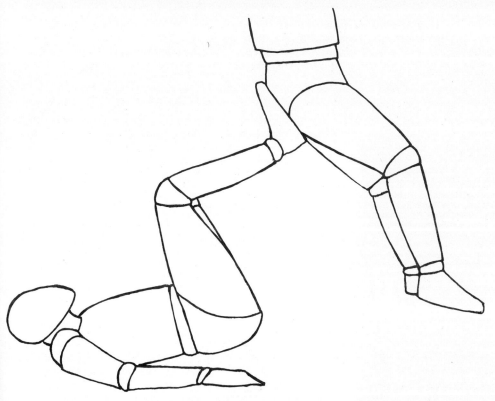

Fig. 8. Buddy push for quadriceps

time. It gives you an excellent lift on the leg to develop the quadricep. You must develop as much flexibility in the quadricep group as possible.

Two additional exercises for the quadriceps are the buddy push (see fig. 8) and the quadriceps stretch (see fig. 9).

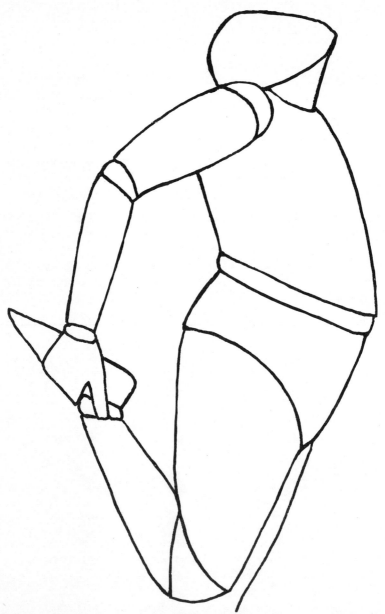

Fig. 9. Quadriceps stretch

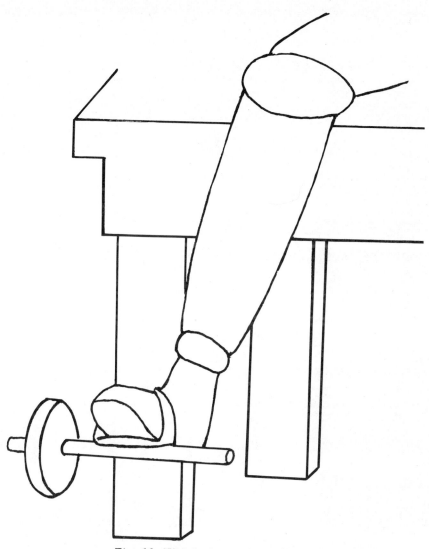

*Fig. 10. Weight boot with weight
on extreme outside of foot*

An area often injured and of prime importance in any conditioning program is the ankle, foot, and supporting musculature. The most common injury to the ankle is the lateral sprain. Knowing this to be so, one should set up an exercise to strengthen the area. The best one for this condition would be to put on a weight boot, placing the weight on the extreme outside end of the bar and raising the weight by everting or turning the foot out and up (see fig. 10).

A good exercise for this area is done by standing with the toes together and heels apart, and raising up on the heels and forcibly turning
the toes out while keeping the heels together. This exercise may have to
be done in partner formation until balance is developed. Flexibility of
the ankle joint is also important; walking 10 to 15 yards every night on
the outside borders of their feet, athletes will develop adequate flexibility
to prevent stretch injuries which result from a sudden force, spraining
the ankle.

No warm-up or exercise program would be complete without strengthening the musculature of the back. Strength here is necessary to prevent
fatigue and to promote both functional posture and great strength.

The best exercise for this area is the stomach rock (see fig. 11). You
may use this exercise either isometrically or isotonically. Lie facedown,
keeping the head, shoulders, arms, chest, and lower extremities clear of
the floor. Arch the back, bringing arms, chest and head up, and raising
legs as high as possible. Return to starting position. Due to the hyper-
extension of the lower back, one may experience soreness the following
day.

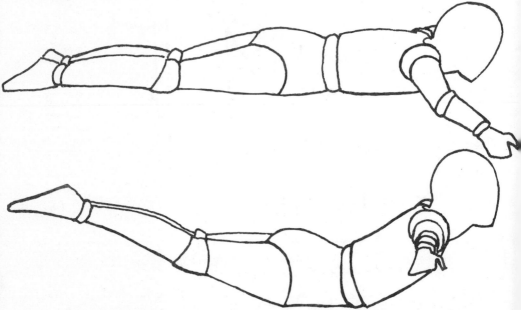

Fig. 11. Stomach rock

There are four other exercises important when warming-up. The first
is the sitting stretch (see fig. 12). Sit, legs spread apart, hands on knees.
Bend forward at waist, extending arms as far forward as possible. Return
to starting position.

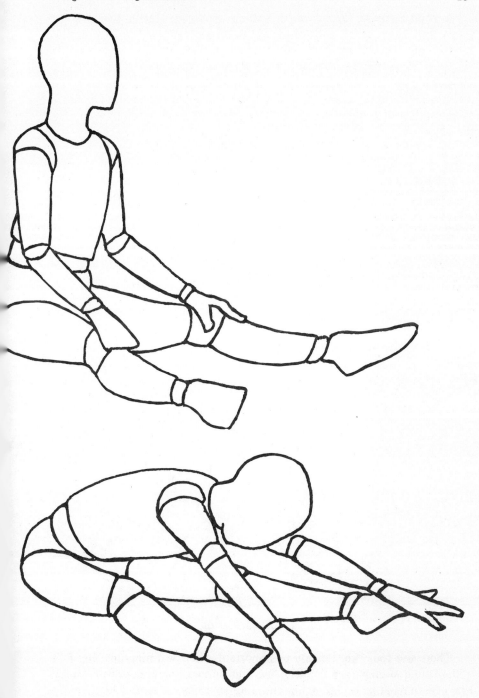

Fig. 12. Sitting stretch

The second is the knee pushup (see fig. 13). Lie on floor, facedown, legs together, knees bent with feet raised off floor, hands on floor under shoulders, palms down. Push upper body off floor until arms are fully extended and body is in straight line from head to knees. Return to starting position.

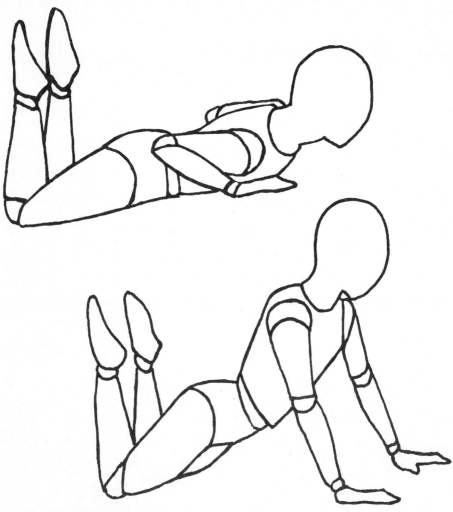

Fig. 13. Knee pushup

The third exercise, already mentioned, is the toe touch (see fig. 14). Stand at attention. Bend trunk forward and down, keeping knees straight, touching fingers to ankles. Bounce and touch fingers to top of feet. Bounce and touch fingers to toes. Return to starting position.

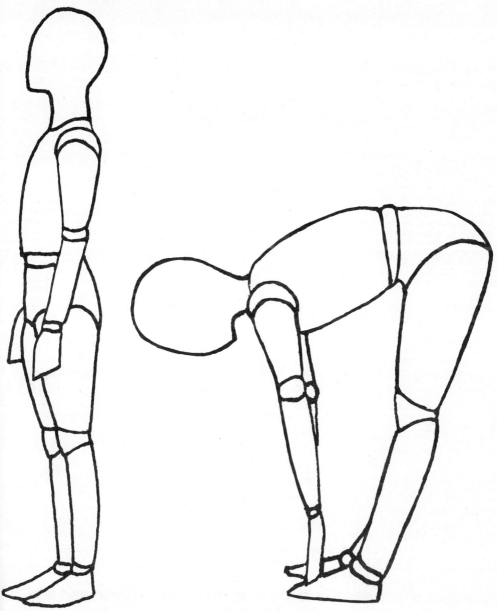

Fig. 14. Toe touch

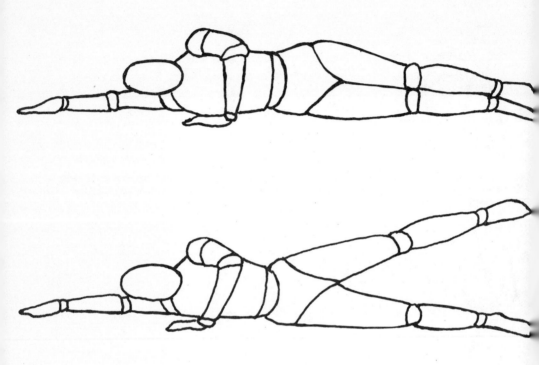

Fig. 15. Leg raiser

The fourth exercise is the leg raiser (see fig. 15). Right side of body on floor, head resting on right arm, lift left leg about 24 inches off floor, then lower it. Do required number of repetitions. Repeat on other side.

In summary, if a boy follows a good warm-up and conditioning session before entering a meet, he will find it will pay dividends. He owes it to himself to be in the best condition when he moves out on that floor to make his run for the blue ribbon.

The Big Ten (see fig. 16) include basic exercises to be practiced daily by child and grown-up alike.

1. *Forward.* Stand with feet apart, raise arms overhead, bending well back; then bend forward, touching the floor with both hands, keeping the legs straight. Start with 8 and work up to 32.

2. *Twist.* In a standing position, extend the arms so they are level with the shoulders, and swing the arms and shoulders in unison from one direction to the other until the muscles of the shoulders and back feel tired.

3. *Turn.* Standing with heels together and arms above head with fingers locked, make a large circle with hands clasped. You should feel the tension of the back, side, and abdominal muscles.

4. *Bend.* From a standing position, move the arms backward and begin to descend into knee-bend position. As you descend lower, move the arms forward while rising.

5. *Stretch.* With the body on the toes and hands, keep legs stiff and arch the back, pushing with hands and legs, and the head turned in toward the knees. Lower the abdomen to the floor (do not touch), head pushed back, and back bent. Start with 12 and work up to 24.

6. *Pull-up.* Grasp a barbell, and while standing erect with legs straight pull the barbell up to the chin and then lower to starting position at thighs.

7. *Press.* Grasp barbell and pull to upper chest and then overhead. Lower to starting position at upper chest.

8. *Row.* With legs straight and body bent forward, pull weight to chest, keeping the back flat and using only the arms.

9. *Lift.* Grasp bar and, with back flat, straighten legs and stand erect with barbell.

10. *Squat.* With bar on shoulders, lower into squat; come up and repeat.

Fig. 16. Big Ten
(Big Ten courtesy of Olympic coach Bob Hoffman)

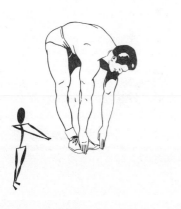 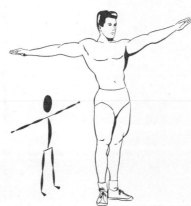

1. Forward   2. Twist

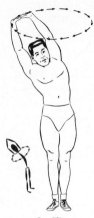

3. Turn

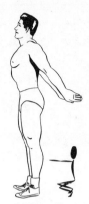

4. Bend

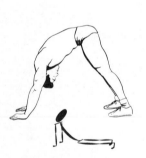

5. Stretch

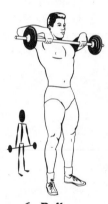

6. Pull-up

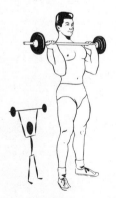

7. Press

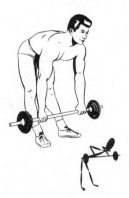

8. Row

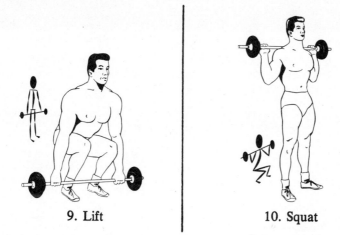

9. Lift   10. Squat

A pre-game workout is necessary for every athlete, and the following series of exercises will prove most valuable in getting the body ready for action.

1. *For the shoulders.* Hold a broomstick overhead, using a wide grip (see fig. 17). Bring it down the back to the hips. Gradually close the space between the hands as muscles warm up.

2. *Front splits.* Assume a wide stance (see fig. 18), one foot forward and the other back. Slide front leg forward, keeping the back foot flat. Hold for a few seconds and repeat on the other leg.

3. *For the neck.* With a weight behind the neck (see fig. 19), bend from the waist as far forward as possible.

4. *Side lunges.* Attach a rope to a support and assume a wide stance. While holding onto the rope, lean back and force the hips forward as you lunge sideward (see fig. 20). Stand and repeat to other side.

5. *Oriental split.* With a wide stance, place hands on floor and slide feet out slowly and work down to the floor as far as possible (see fig. 21).

6. *For the ankles.* With heel on floor, force ball of foot against a support, keeping leg straight (see fig. 22).

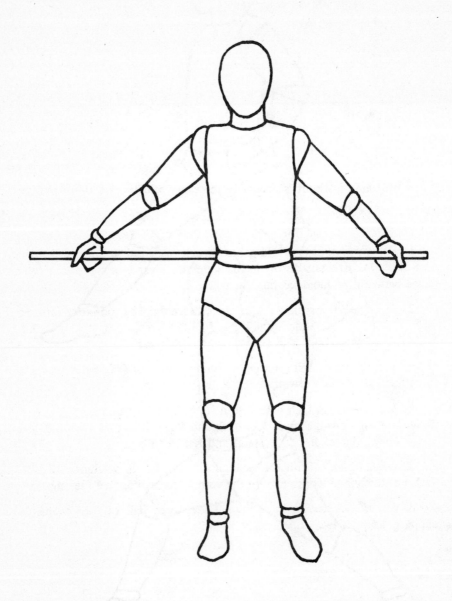

Fig. 17. For the shoulders

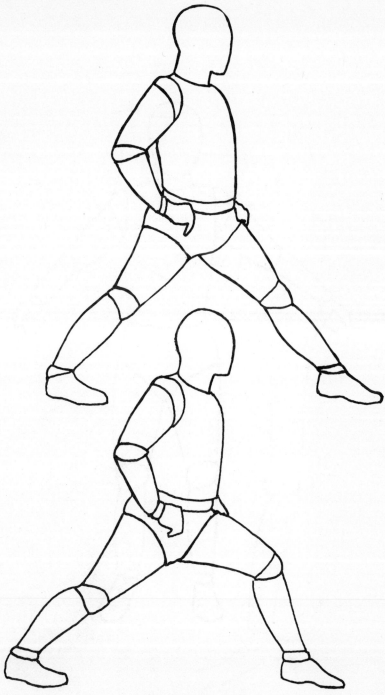

Fig. 18. Front split

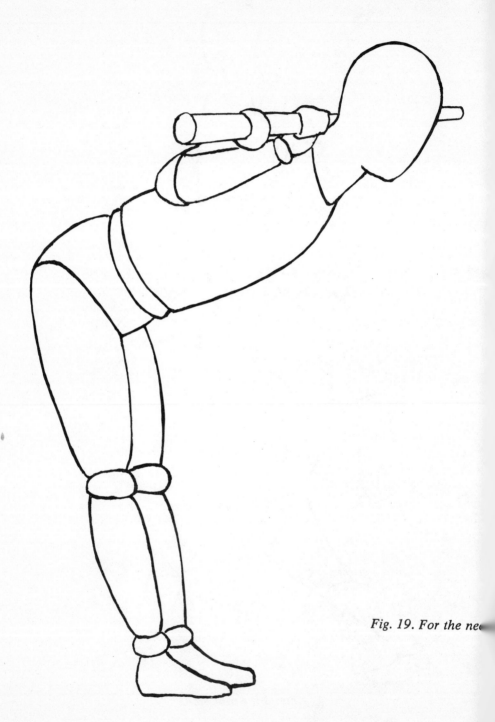

Fig. 19. For the ne

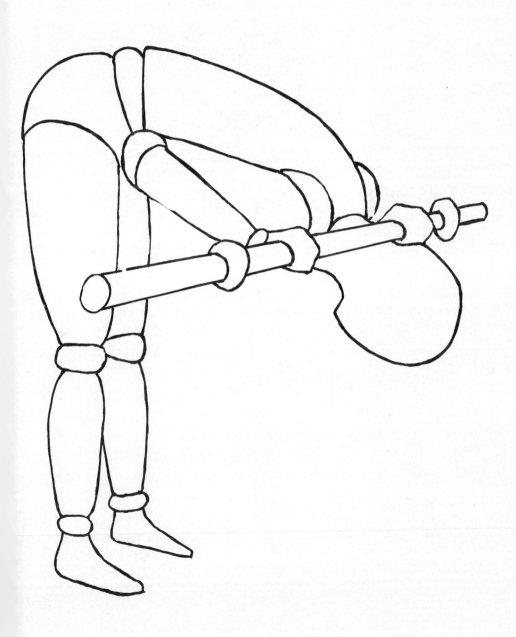

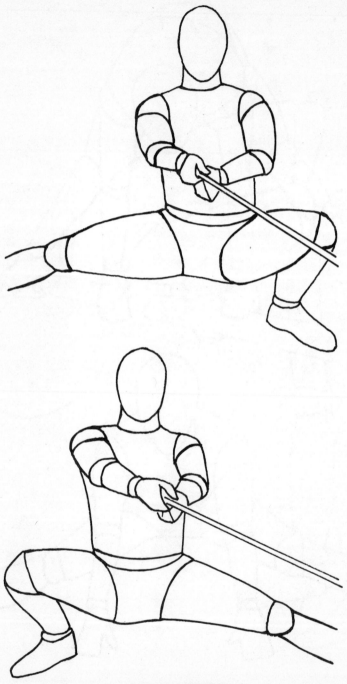

Fig. 20. Side lunge

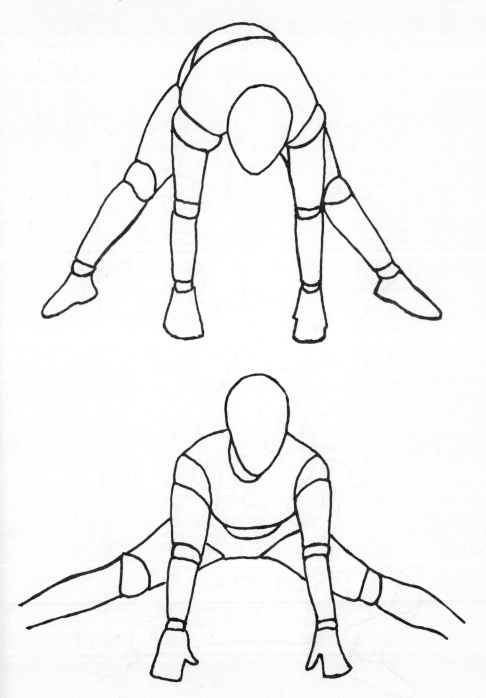

Fig. 21. Oriental split

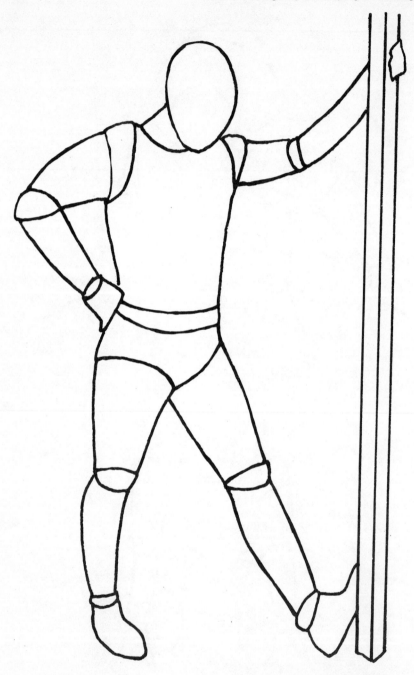

Fig. 22. For the ankles

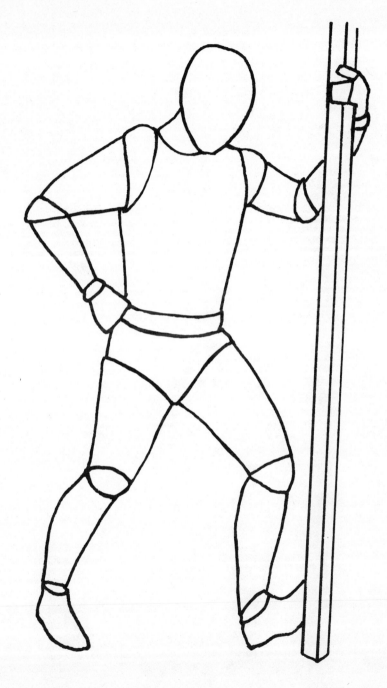

BASIC EXERCISES

"Doctor, which exercise will help me most?"

This is a frequently asked question and very difficult to answer. We all need a general exercise program, but there are special exercises that will help some more than others. Sometimes exercises must be tailored to you like an article of clothing. Some of us need exercises designed for our anatomical strengths and weaknesses (for example, poor posture, one leg shorter than the other).

There are a number of excellent circulatory exercises designed by qualified men in the field of physical education. One of the oldest and best exercises is running in place (see fig. 23). Stand erect, extending both elbows parallel to the floor, and run in place, bringing the right knee up, then the left, as high as you can. Beginners should start with 30 counts or steps. Add 10 more counts each day until you reach 60 counts.

The *10-hop* is another fine exercise (see fig. 24). Place your hands on your hips; then hop on your right foot for a count of 10; repeat on your left foot. Then spread your legs as far as possible and hop on both feet for a count of 10. From an erect position, hop to the left on your left foot for a count of 10, and hop back into position for the same count. Repeat on right foot, jumping to the right.

An excellent exercise to follow the above is called the *ventilation* and *circulation exercise* and calls for a good, deep breath (see fig. 25). Standing erect, take in a good, deep breath, blow it all out, and take in a second, larger one—hold it. Bring your arms up to a forward position, at the same time rising on your toes and pressing down hard on the balls of your feet, so that you feel a pressure on your ankles, calves, and thighs. Then slowly return to original position while exhaling. Repeat exercise 6 times.

There is an exercise I was taught as a boy, and it was used at that time to prevent tuberculosis and to try to develop the chest and lungs. We fail to realize how important it is to expand the upper part of the lungs underneath the clavicles of the first and second ribs, to open up the chest and air sacs of the lungs. The exercise that follows is the best treatment for the spine, ribs, and chest, and puts the ribs through their normal range. It has done more good for more people, including myself, and I have demonstrated it to boys and girls in over fifty countries. The exercise is called *thumbs up* (see figs. 26a, 26b, 26c). Standing erect, place your arms behind your back, interlacing your fingers so that they are pushing outward, pushing your thumbs (about 2 inches apart) up your spine as far as possible, one on each side of the spine. Force your arms down toward the floor as far as they will go, turning your hands over so that the thumbs are turning in against your lower back and buttocks. When you finish, your palms should be facing the floor. You must not let go of your fingers; it might be necessary to release the first or second, but try to hold the last two fingers and palms facedown. From this position, take a deep breath, getting all the air you can while rising on your toes (a slight, bouncing movement); then try to take in a little more, as you start walking with long steps, all the while holding your breath. Start by taking at least 10 steps, and increase this up to at least 30, holding your breath up to one full minute. In this position, you have extended your chest, opened it up wide, letting the air circulate under your clavicles and under the area of the first and second ribs. You have stretched your spine and, with the expansion of the lungs, elevated all of your ribs, putting them through their normal physiological motion. This is a good exercise to do on your way to school, if both hands are free and you are walking. It develops and brings the chest up and gives that excellent feeling of well-being and warmth by circulating the oxygen through your entire body. It is also excellent for improving the posture.

Isometric exercises are of a different nature but are equally as valuable as strenuous ones. Designed to build muscle and strength, they consist of flexing one muscle against another. They are exercises that can be done on the way to school or when you are at your books. When you're a bit tired, you can do these exercises right in your chiar, anytime, either from a sitting or standing position.

This first isometric exercise is called the *press* (see fig. 27). Stand erect, clamp hands close to your chest, palms together, and press hands hard, holding for a count of 6 seconds (say "1,001, 1,002, 1,003"). It is very important to have a good count. If counting aloud, try not to lose any air while you are pushing. Repeat three times; then drop your hands in front of your abdomen, press them together, and hold tight for a count of 6.

The *tug-of-war* (see fig. 28) is another isometric exercise. Stand erect, bring your arms close to your chest, clasping fingers of your left and right hands; pull as hard as you can trying to pull your fingers apart and hold for a count of 6. Repeat exercise in the same manner with the hands held in front of your abdomen.

To do the *elbow bender* (see fig. 29), extend your left palm upward with your elbow close to your body; place right hand over the left, clasp-it snugly, forcefully attempting to curl the left arm upward while resisting with the right arm. Hold for a count of 6 seconds. Change positions, extending the right arm, palm up, with the elbow close to the body, placing the left hand over the right. Repeat once if desired (hold, rest, repeat).

Fourth in the series is the *pull* (see fig. 30). Standing erect, place your right hand over your left, which is being held against the small of the back. Pull at the muscles of your right arm, attempting to resist the strength of the muscles of the left for a count of 6; rest and repeat. Reverse position and pull at left arm for a count of 6; rest and repeat.

The fifth exercise is the *overhead stretch* (see fig. 31). Standing erect, pull your hands overhead, stand on your toes, and stretch as high as you can to the count of 6.

The last in the series is the *upper-back exercise* (see fig. 32). Put the palms of your hands in front of your chest, the right against the left, and firmly push and hold to a count of 6. Take a deep breath, pull as hard as you can for a count of 6, relax for a count of 6, and then press again for the same count.

Section II

BASIC HEALTH

THE BASIC PHYSICAL

In sports training or weight lifting, regardless of age, it is advisable for the young athlete to have a physical examination, including some laboratory work. I am aware that it is impossible to do extensive examinations in many areas, but a basic, physical examination, including simple tests, should be done. If abnormal conditions are present, they should be investigated.

For instance, the examination for a boy entering weight training and weight lifting should consist of having him undress to allow proper inspection of his body for posture, one leg shorter than the other, a curvature, level shoulders, spondylitis, swayback—anything particularly wrong with his spine as he stands up before a mirror. Is the distance between the earlobe and the shoulder the same on both sides? (Allow the boy to see this while you are examining him.) The next procedure would be to take his blood pressure in both arms while he is standing, sitting, and lying down. Administer a basic stress test (see fig. 33). Using a sturdy bench or chair about 15-17 inches high, have the patient do the following four-count movement: place right foot on bench; bring left foot up and stand; lower right foot to floor; lower left foot to floor. Repeat movement 30 times a minute for two minutes. Have patient rest on chair or bench for two minutes. Take pulse for 30 seconds. Double the count to get the rate per minute. Repeat test once every two weeks and compare pulse records.

Check his breathing, his respiratory rate—does he take a good, deep breath? What is his chest expansion? What about his height and weight? Is he underweight? overweight? Is he the normal weight for his age? Check his eyes. He may be nearsighted. Don't overlook refractive tests in your examination of his eyes.

Check his throat. Is he subject to colds? Does he have a sinus infection? Are his muscles comparatively well developed? What about his thyroid? Are his neck and thyroid visibly enlarged? Does he have a choking sensation? Listen to his chest; are there any rales in his chest? If his chest expansion is normal, there shouldn't be.

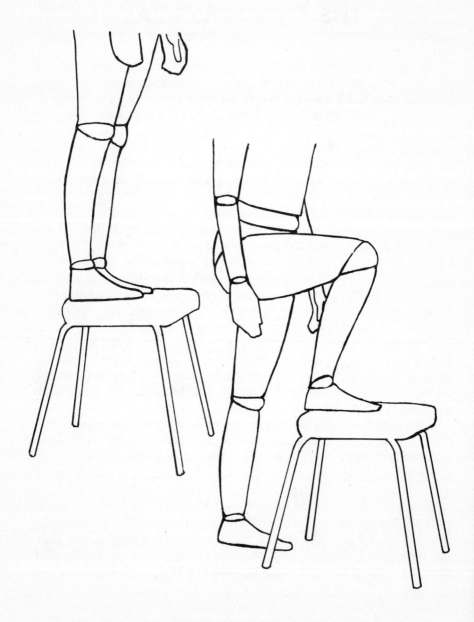

Fig. 33. Basic stress test

Check the individual's reflexes. See that he has a good patella reflex on each side, that his Achilles tendon is normal, that his radials are normal, that he can focus his eyes well on the end of your finger. Hold out his hands and see if he has a tremor. Blindfold him and see if he can touch his nose with his right hand and left, and have him lie down and see if he can put his right heel on his left big toe and his left heel on his right big toe. These are some tests that will show you something about his coordination and his reflexes.

Check his nose and nasal passages. Transilluminate his sinuses—is there any thickening in this area? This is somewhat difficult to judge because of the age of the boy, the amount of sinuses he has, and their development. Does he have a guttural tone? Does his nose plug up? If his nose is plugged up a great part of the time, does he have an allergy? Is it worse at any one time of the year than another, or does it remain the same? He may have an allergy, and you should take a culture from the boy's nose. These bacteria can be killed and an autogenous vaccine made and tested. Sometimes we find the boy is allergic to his own infection. If this is true, an autogenous vaccine can be devised to help this individual. It is also good to discover if he feels worse, or if his nose or head plugs up if he eats any particular kind of food or if he has been in different parts of the country. This is not a thorough examination but it is adequate.

It's well to take an x-ray of the boy's chest, do a urinalysis on him, and take a simple blood count to check that his clotting time is normal. If he is a black boy, I would recommend doing a Schilling count. In the urinalysis, check for albumin, sugar, and look for casts. If possible, check for a history of urinary problems; check to see that his bowels move regularly. When the boy is undressed, check for a hernia, that he has two testicles, that they are in the scrotum, and that he does not have an undescended testicle. Does he have any rashes or skin disease of any type? Test for V.D.

If you do find that the boy has a history of rheumatic fever, or an irregularity in his pulse, or his blood pressure is not what it should be, do an electrocardiogram. It may reveal a heart defect or irregularity. It may also be necessary to have the boy undergo a treadmill stress test (see fig. 34).

An individual with a heart problem should have a stress test before he enters extensive athletic programs. The individual walks on the treadmill, the angle of elevation and speed increasing so he has to walk faster. The pitch is also raised, making a more uphill walk. While this is being done, a blood-pressure cuff on his arm checks his pressure constantly, and an electrocardiogram machine records his heartbeat. His pulse is also monitored as the workload increases. A clothespin is put on his nose so that he breathes oxygen through a tube in his mouth, and we measure the amount of oxygen he is breathing in, and the amount of carbon dioxide he is putting out. It might be well to check his blood's lactic-acid level.

The stress test is not a simple one. It's a test which is rather expensive and takes considerable time, equipment and energy to do, but it's very worthwhile and important to know the patient's ability to compete in active sports.

A final reminder—when examining the various muscles and groups of muscles in the body, it is well to use the following charts as a guideline. Indicate where the most work is needed to develop the muscles for the strength used in the sport in which the athlete will be participating; check his range of motion (see figs. 35 through 38). Be sure to check bone structure and joint movement. Look for flat feet, good arches, corns, ingrown toenails, fungus of the feet, plantar warts, and general, painful areas about the knees, back, neck, shoulders, and for headaches.

Pre-Season Screening Tests
of Strength and Flexibility

Rating Scale

Normal—4
Fair—3
Poor—2
Excessively weak or tight—1
Current injury does not permit test—0
(F—flexibility) (S—strength)

	Right		Left		Comments
	S	F	S	F	
A. Tests from Supine Position					
1. Shoulder Flexors (S&F)					
2. Shoulder Extensors (S&F)					
3. Shoulder Adductors (S&F)					
4. Internal Rotators (S&F)					
5. External Rotators (S&F)					
6. Abdominals (S&F)					
7. Dorsi Flexion at Ankle (F)					
8. Inversion at Ankle (F)					
B. Tests from Sitting Position					
1. Groin (adductors) (F)					
2. Hamstrings (F)					
3. Low Back (F)					
4. Biceps (S&F)					
5. Triceps (S&F)					
6. Wrist Flexors (S&F)					
7. Wrist Extensors (S&F)					
C. Tests from Prone Position					
1. Quadriceps (S&F)					
2. Hamstrings (S)					
3. Erector Spinar (S)					
4. Hip Extension (S)					
D. Tests from Standing Position					
1. Hip Flexors (S&F)					
2. Gastrocnemius (S)					
3. Anterior Tibialis (S)					
4. Evertors at Ankle (F&S)					
5. Longitudinal Arch (flat feet) (S)					

Fig. 35. Pre-season screening tests
of strength and flexibility

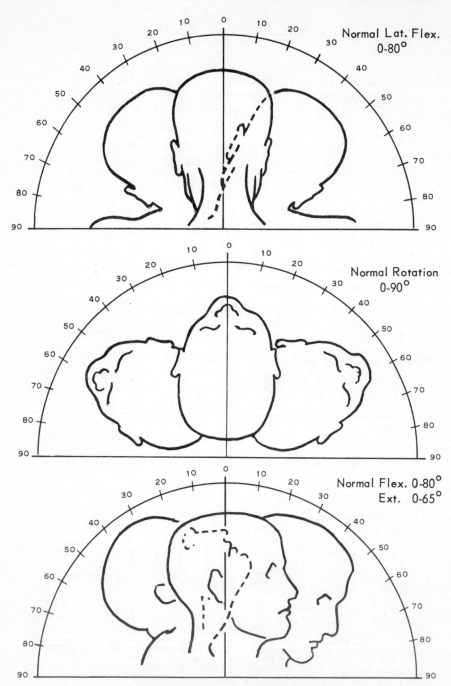

*Fig. 36. Range of motion and strength evaluation
(cervical musculature)*

Fig. 37. Range of motion test
for lower extremity

1. Anatomical position is starting position. Range is measured with cauda as 0°, cranium as 180°. Rotating motions are from the midsagittal plane as 0° to lateral plane as 180°.

2. All ranges are expressed as passive range of motion. Check muscle chart attached for limitations caused by tightness, weakness, spasm, or contracture.

3. The scale is divided into units of 10°. Range of motion is recorded by filling in area of range directly on attached sketch with date and examiner's initial.

4. Use of same sheet for subsequent tests is recorded in same color and dated accordingly.

5. Retrogression is marked by diagonal lines over area of previous test and dated.

6. If position is other than in sketch, indicate S for supine, P for prone.

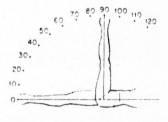

Hip

Flexion (straight knee)	0-90
Flexion (bent knee)	0-115-125
Extension	0- 10- 15
Extension and lumbar- spine	0- 15- 45

Limitations
Flexion (straight knee)

	L		R	
	Fl.	Ext.	Fl.	Ext.
1				
2				

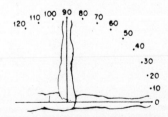

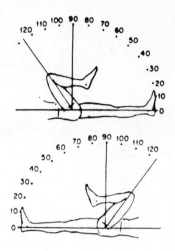

Flexion (bent knee)

	L		R	
	Fl.	Ext.	Fl.	Ext.
1				
2				

Extension

	L		R	
	Ext.	E & L	Ext.	E & L
1				
2				

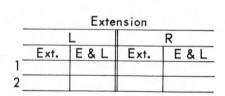

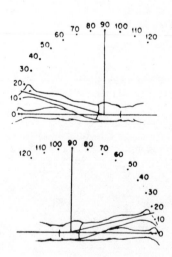

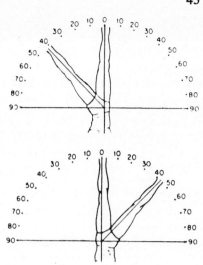

Hip

Abduction	0-45
Adduction	45- 0

Limitations

	L		R	
	Abd.	Add.	Abd.	Add.
1				
2				

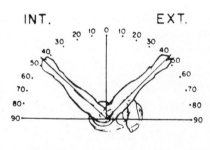

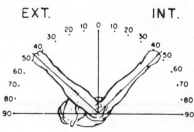

Hip (bent knee prone)

External rotation	0-45
Internal rotation	0-45

Limitations

	L		R	
	Int.	Ext.	Int.	Ext.
1				
2				

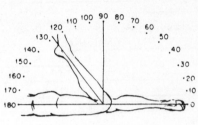

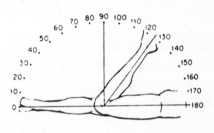

Knee

Flexion (prone)	0-120-130
Extension	130-120- 0

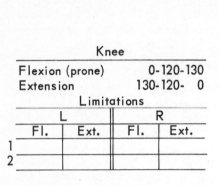

	Limitations			
	L		R	
	Fl.	Ext.	Fl.	Ext.
1				
2				

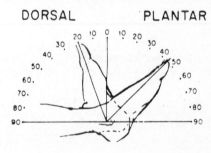

DORSAL   PLANTAR

Ankle

Flexion	0-20
Extension	0-45

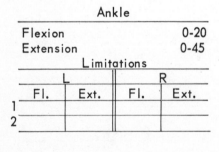

	Limitations			
	L		R	
	Fl.	Ext.	Fl.	Ext.
1				
2				

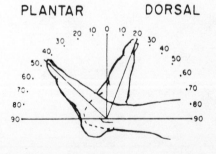

PLANTAR   DORSAL

Foot	
Eversion	0-25
Inversion	0-35

Limitations			
L		R	
Ev.	Inv.	Ev.	Inv.
1			
2			

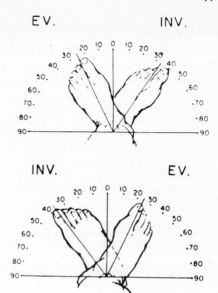

EV.　　　　　　INV.

INV.　　　　　　EV.

Fig. 38. Range of motion test
for upper extremity

1. Anatomical position is starting position. Range is measured with cauda as 0°, cranium as 180°. Rotating motions are from the midsagittal plane as 0° to lateral plane as 180°.

2. All ranges are expressed as passive range of pain free motion. Check muscle chart attached for limitations caused by tightness, weakness, spasm, or contracture.

3. The scale is divided into units of 10°. Range of motion is recorded by filling in area of range directly on attached sketch with date and examiner's initial.

4. Use of same sheet for subsequent tests is recorded in same color and dated accordingly.

5. Retrogression is marked in red and dated.

6. If position is other than in sketch, indicate S for supine, P for prone.

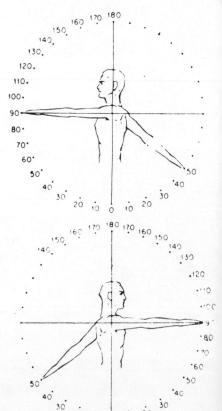

Shoulder

Flexion	0-90
Flexion and rotation of scapula	90-180
Extension and rotation of scapula	180-90
Extension	90-50

Limitations

	L		R	
	Fl.	Ext.	Fl.	Ext.
1				
2				

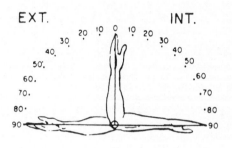

Shoulder Rotation

Elbow flexed	90°
External rotation	0-90
Internal rotation	0-90

Limitations

	L			R	
	Int.	Ext.		Int.	Ext.
1					
2					

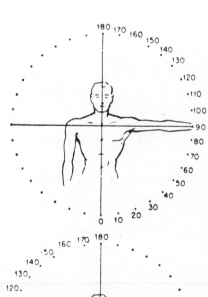

Shoulder

Abduction	0-90
Abduction and rotation of scapula	90-180
Adduction and rotation of scapula	180-90
Adduction	90-0

Limitations

	L			R	
	Abd.	Add.		Abd.	Add.
1					
2					

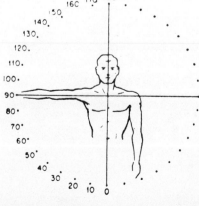

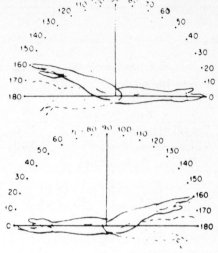

Elbow

Flexion	0-145-160
Extension	160-145-0

Limitations

	L			R	
	Flex.	Ext.		Flex.	Ext.
1					
2					

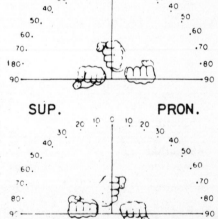

Radio-ulnar

Pronation	0-90
Supination	0-90

Limitations

	L			R	
	Sup.	Pron.		Sup.	Pron.
1					
2					

Wrist (flexion)

Dorsal flexion	0-70
Volar flexion	0-90

Limitations

	L			R	
	Dor.	Vol.	Dor.	Vol.
1				
2				

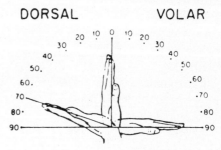

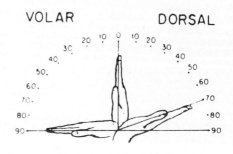

Wrist

Abduction	0-25
Adduction	0-55-65

Limitations

	L			R	
	Rad.	Uln.	Rad.	Uln.
1				
2				

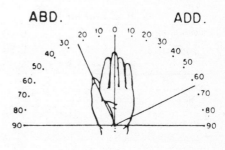

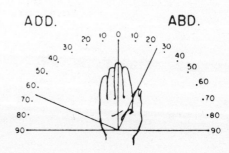

BLOOD PRESSURE

Having studied athletes for many years, it is the opinion of the author that every athlete participating in a national championship, world's championship, or Olympics should have his blood pressure taken before he goes into competition. If his pressure is high, the check should be repeated because an irregularity may be caused by the excitement of the competition.

There is nothing difficult about taking blood pressure. A mature individual who trains alone, or who is nowhere near a doctor, coach, or trainer, can take his own blood pressure; all he needs is a blood-pressure kit. I have found that 95 percent of all people can learn to take their own blood pressure accurately and correctly, even 10-year-old children, within fifteen to twenty minutes.

In any sports program, it is imperative that we not send a boy with hypertension out onto the floor to lift. We should know what his blood pressure is, and, if he is injured, we should know that, too; it is possible his injury is causing his hypertension.

Blood pressure should be taken while the athlete is standing, sitting, and lying down. The pressure will vary in these three positions. If the pressure is high in an individual, it might be well to have him rest or walk away, leaving the cuff on his arm; then have him sit and gradually retake it. You might have to take it several times because the excitement may increase the pressure, making it much higher than it normally is, as happens in some athletes.

An excellent time to check these individuals' blood pressure is when they are waiting to be weighed in. The weighing-in process takes a considerable period of time prior to the lifting. Before or after that, there is always a physician on duty, and individual pressures should be taken at the time of the contest.

DIET

In this year of Olympic sesquicentennial celebration, many of us will be taking the time to return to the past, to rediscover our heritage, and admire those men and women who made this country great. One wonders, in those days of old, just how people survived the trials and tribulations they did without the help of doctors and the knowledge we have today about good nutrition.

Of the many topics of importance when discussing sports and medicine, good nutrition rates high on the list of coaches, trainers, physicians and athletes. I recently reviewed a book on just that subject, and it discussed carbohydrates, fats, protein, vitamins, and minerals. But do we know as much about them, in our modern times, as we think we do? And how much more is there to learn?

By now it is common knowledge that fad diets do not work, nor are they healthy. An athlete needs a balanced diet—three good meals a day and even a snack in the evening. Calories? They're important, and one's daily intake should depend on his weight, size, and how many calories the athlete will expend during his workouts. I asked Bruce Jenner, winner of the World Champion Decathlon and now training for the Montreal Olympics, about his daily food intake. He eats three balanced meals a day, and if he feels so inclined, has a small snack at night. He's 6 foot, 2 inches tall and weighs between 190 and 195 lbs. It is at this weight that that he functions his best, and he realizes the importance of maintaining it.

What exactly does a balanced diet consist of? We know the body needs protein, fats, carbohydrates, minerals and vitamins. These come from meat, fish, vegetables, fruit, cereals, and dairy products. Let's be more specific. We get a supply of protein and fat (we do need some fat) from meat, fish, milk, cheese, yogurt and other dairy products. Cereals also provide protein and carbohydrates (the latter supply energy); oats, corn, wheat, buckwheat, rye, barley, and wild and brown rice supply these, as well as the B vitamins. By the way, when taking antibiotics, it is wise to eat yogurt to replace the body's necessary bacteria being destroyed by drugs. Nuts from all sections of the country are also a fine source of nutrition.

Fresh vegetables and fruit are abundant sources of vitamins. Citrus fruits are an excellent source of vitamin C, and if we include fresh vegetables and fruit in our diet, we will have created a nutritional food pattern for our bodies. If one eats a balanced diet, vitamin supplements are unnecessary. A note on additives: read labels carefully, taking note of those chemicals which may be harmful to your health, especially red dye added for coloring.

SINUS PROBLEMS

A good percentage of the athletes at the Winter Olympics in Innsbruck developed colds, the flu, bronchitis, disturbances in their middle ear (some had runny ears); others felt a blocked-up sensation, and their heads felt like a piece of wood. This was accompanied by a headache, stuffy nose, some difficulty in breathing, nasal drip, a hacking cough, and nausea, all caused by one condition—stuffed up or infected sinuses.

The first consideration for the Olympic lifter is not to use any drugs noted on the O.I.C. forbidden list. This list is distributed to everyone, and to have an athlete use a drug that is on this list is just plain stupid. As president of the Medical Committee for the International Federation of Weightlifting at the Munich Olympics, it was necessary to call a drug hearing meeting on two occasions. Both individuals had a positive reaction in the urine—they had taken a forbidden drug.

This was unfortunate and very embarrassing for the individuals, as well as for their physicians, coaches and trainers; there's no excuse for this. There are numerous drugs that might be substituted for those on the list, and certainly a report should be made to the O.I.C. prior to competition so a decision can be made.

Treatment for an acute sinus condition and stuffed-up nose is as follows: the patient lies on his back, his head extended out over the end of the table so that the crown of the head is well below the level of the table, and the head is lower than the throat. With the patient in this position, place four drops of an astringent nose drop into each nostril, and then gently massage the entire triangular area between the nostrils and the eye.

After three minutes have the patient rise, clear his head, and then resume his original position and repeat the treatment two more times. There are three turbinates in each nostril, and each has to be shrunk. The bottom one must be shrunk before the middle and upper can be cleared. That is why it is necessary to perform the procedure three times, to get an opening, reduce the swelling and clear the debris from the nose at the entrance to the sinuses.

When the sinuses are clear, the patient should put lukewarm saline in the cup of his hand and sniff it up into his nostrils. This has a tendency to dissolve and clear out debris. Now that the patient's nose is open and

57

he can breathe, he should lie on his back with his head on a pillow. Hyperextend his neck, working it in a slow, rhythmic motion. Have him rotate his neck to the right with extension, then rotate to the left with extension, trying to clear out anv areas of congestion or soreness in this pumpinglike manner.

At the base of the skull lies a group of muscles known as the *rectus capitis major* and *minor,* eight small muscles attaching the first two vertebrae to the skull (see fig. 39). Due to the headache or feeling of stuffiness the person has because of his sinus condition, he walks many times as though he were walking on eggs, and this group of muscles play a part in holding the head so rigid that the muscles become spastic, which interferes with the drainage from the skull and brain.

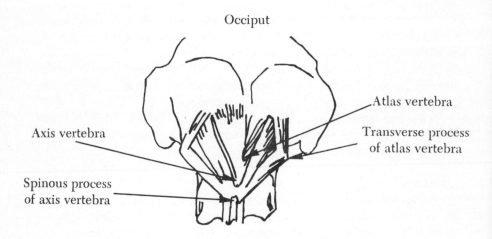

Fig. 39. Rectus capitis major and minor

By putting the hand at the base of the skull, putting an extension on the head, and putting pressure up into the area between the occipital vertebrae, one can produce a relaxation of these muscles, and on many occasions in one or two minutes a severe headache will disappear.

I saw a boy suffering all of these difficulties at 4:00 P.M. knowing that weigh-in time was at 6:00 P.M. He was given the aforementioned treatment and then I exerted some deep pressure with rotary motion over the frontal sinuses and also down over the ethmoids in between the eyes and nose, pressing on both the right and left sides, trying to produce some motion between those bones for greater drainage. By 6:00 P.M., when he weighed in, his head was clear and he felt like a different person. He was able to make his run for the gold.

EARACHE AND RUNNY EAR

Shortly after arriving at the national championships, I got a call from a trainer saying that one of his athletes had an earache. He had difficulty hearing, and he was restless. I found that the athlete had an otitis media infection, and the eardrum was probably ruptured and draining.

There are any number of drugs used in this case, but we must be concerned for a person who may be allergic to certain drugs, especially penicillin. The one treatment that has proved more valuable to us in this case than any other is the system a group of Upstate New York pediatricians use. They administer 1 gram per day dosage of penicillin. I have followed their system and found it has a remarkable effect in curbing recurring middle-ear infections. An alternate, low dose of sulfisoxazole may be given, but penicillin seems to be the best available drug for the prevention of recurrent ear infection or otitis media in young athletes. In addition, 1 gram per day of penicillin administered to small children or infants is usually increased to 2 to 3 grams, depending on the size and weight of the individual.

THE BLUE RIBBON
BOWEL MOVEMENT

Did you have a bowel movement today? You say, "No, not for several days." Well, you are certainly not in the best shape to grab that blue ribbon. This is definitely not a good position to be in on the day of the competition.

When athletes go to an international competition, they usually experience a change in food, water, and, many times, weather. If it is hot, they are apt to become considerably dehydrated, losing a lot of their body fluids. Their habits are irregular, and facilities not being always adequate or available, they may miss a bowel movement for a day or maybe as many as four or five days. The individual feels toxic and not well—not sick, but not at his best—and when you find this condition, the most important thing is to prevent its happening again.

When I'm with a team, I like to get to know these boys all well enough individually to ask personal questions about their excretory functions. Is their voiding O.K.? Are they able to urinate? Have they had normal bowel movements? Is there any bleeding? Any itching or any irritation around the rectum?

The person who goes several days without a bowel movement may have a very hard stool, and he may tear or cut a membrane. This fissure can, in turn, break and form what we call a pocket later on, and, as it extends outward, this pocket will form a bulge beneath this membrane with the veins on each side of the rectum. We then say he has internal hemorrhoids; if they break through the skin surface, coming out, they become external hemorrhoids. From this the athlete may develop an opening above and then, from some infection, break through to the outside of the rectum in the skin—now he has a rectal fistula, which is then, depending on its location, somewhat difficult to take care of.

This can be avoided by making certain that the athlete has a daily bowel movement. There are a few ways to deal with the problem. One product I have found very beneficial is called Metamucil, which adds bulk. If the individual is having a bowel problem, he should take a teaspoon of Metamucil in a glass of water (8 ounces), followed by a second glass of water. This should be taken in the evening after dinner, or a couple of hours before going to bed. If the condition is severe, he should take two teaspoons of Metamucil and then follow each one with a glass of water (four glasses of water in all—about a liter). For this condition, he should also have some prune juice for breakfast or prunes in the evening. We try to cure it with natural food, but, if it's necessary, we resort to some chemical activity. Usually this will take care of the matter if it has not become too severe.

Now the athlete will feel great for the competition. Instead of lifting 5 lbs. or 2 kilos less, he'll lift 5 lbs. or approximately 2 kilos more and probably win the meet.

There are many suppositories that can be used for rectal irritation and to soften the stool and cut down the irritation.

Get in the good habit of having a bowel movement every morning, usually about the same time. It will become a habit and will take care of a multitude of your problems in sports competition and through the rest of your life.

"OH! MY ACHING BACK!"

This club is the largest and unorganized, with members everywhere. In my worldwide traveling, one of the first questions asked of me is, "What's new in treating back problems?" My answer is to ask yourself the following questions, and from them I think we can come up with solutions to some back problems.

How does your back condition affect you? How long have you had it? Is it getting worse? Can you stand in one place for a long period on both feet, or do you have to stand on one foot and then the other, alternating as time passes? Does your problem keep you awake at night? Which is more comfortable to you—a hard bed or a soft one? Have you been in any automobile accidents, or had falls or injuries, especially ski injuries? Does your pain come on suddenly or slowly? If you cough or sneeze, does the pain increase? Give yourself a posture test. Can you stand straight with your head, back and heels up against the wall (see fig. 40)? Does your back condition usually clear up quickly, or does it take a long time? Do you have treatment of some type or medication for it? Have you had a myelogram? In this test a dye is injected into the spinal canal, congenital defects? Have you ever had polio? Do you have any birth defects?

Have you had x-rays taken of your back? When I say x-rays of your back, I'm speaking of the lower back, and views from front to back, a side view, a right and left oblique (three-quarter views), a spot film right where the last vertebra (the fifth) joins the sacrum (which lies between the two sacroiliacs), a Ferguson angle film for spondylitis, and last, but not least, a standing x-ray of your lower back, extending from the top of the trochanters up to approximately the twelve dorsal vertebrae in order to measure the length of the spine and look for any tilt in the pelvis. If you have had this done, and all was reported as negative, have you had any surgery on your back, legs, or knees? Do you have any and x-rays arc taken. The dye can be traced as it flows into areas of the root canals or may be blocked out of areas by a ruptured disc. This is done to determine if there is a ruptured intervertebral disc. Do you have sacroiliac pain? Is it on the left side or on the right? Does it extend down your legs? Have you had any numbness in your foot, pain down your leg, especially on the outside of your leg between the knee and the ankle, or numbness along the outside of your foot or on top? Have you noticed

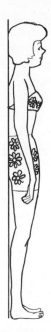

Fig. 40. Posture test

any weakness in your big toe when you go to press it down? Do you have the strength to push it down and raise it up under pressure? Have you noticed that you have a tendency to be awkward or to trip? If you are in your bare feet, do you catch and bump your toes? Stand before a mirror; is one of your shoulders higher than the other? Is the tip of your shoulder nearer to the tip of your ear on one side of your body than on the other? Is your head tilted to the right or left side? This is what makes the measurement of the distance between your earlobe and your shoulder look longer or shorter. When standing, does one arm hang lower than the other? Have you taken medication for pain? If so, how long? One dose or over several days? Has this condition caused you to go to bed and rest? Have you ever been told that you have arthritis? Do you have trouble getting up from a chair to a standing position? Do you have to reach out with your hands when you are sitting in a captain's chair, and grab the arms of the chair and pull yourself up and out, or can you push yourself up out of the chair with your legs? Can you walk well once you get up, or are you tilted to the right or the left? Is it almost impossible for you to straighten up into an erect position and stand tall?

Does one leg tire more easily than the other? Are your leg and thigh smaller on one side than on the other? Can you stoop over, say for a half an hour while you are pulling weeds or picking strawberries or any function where you are working down on the ground, or do you have to get down onto your knees? Does your job require the use of your right arm or right hand or left arm or left hand, causing it to be larger than the other? Does your back hurt in any particular place? Can you put your finger on the area? Does it hurt to ride your bicycle? Does your back hurt if you have to ride a long distance in a car? If you sit in school on a hard seat, does your back hurt when you get up? Does your back feel worse in the morning, at noon, or later in the afternoon?

What have you done for your back? What kind of treatments have you had—hot or cold packs, exercise, physical therapy, electrical stimulation, traction, both rhythmic and sustained, ultrasonic (sound wave) treatment, diathermy, whirlpool, massage and manipulation or corrective adjustment?

It has been my experience over a great many years to ask these questions of a patient with a backache or pain and, after a survey of them and doing the usual laboratory work, find that the patient does not have a tumor of the spine, that his myelogram is negative, and there is no protrusion of the intervertebral disc. It is then discovered that one of the patient's legs is shorter than the other. It is not uncommon to find ¾ of an inch or an inch difference, but the usual variance is approximately 5/16 of an inch.

When I was young and played ball, it was discovered that I had this condition. I was being scouted by major-league teams; it was observed that I could run well in one direction on the side of the short leg, but on the side of the long leg I moved not nearly as well because I lost a half a step on the start.

I was so impressed by this that I made a study of it. Applying the study to athletes worldwide, I've found many of them with this condition, which I discovered could be brought about by injury, in addition to irregular growth patterns. Today some physicians put staples at the joint (growth center) on the shorter leg to stimulate that leg to grow more for balance. This is done to the youngster at puberty, before these joints, the growth centers, are closed.

This postural imbalance can be mechanically corrected and the back restored to a normal position and the rotation taken out; this is done by building up the one shoe. In the meantime, the patient should get physical therapy, especially rhythmic traction and sustained, and a special exercise program worked out. After he's worn the shoe for anywhere from a few days to a couple of weeks (depending on the case), x-ray him again with his shoes on to check the balance; when that balance has been arrived at, the patient will become free of pain, his backache will disappear, and he will no longer be a candidate for the "OH! MY ACHING BACK!" club. (For more detailed information, see the following chapter.)

THE LOST CHAMPIONSHIP

Every athlete strives for perfection. He dreams of an undefeated season, a district championship, a Player-of-the-Year Award—all very admirable goals, certainly. However, to accomplish this, every aspect of the athlete's health must be checked; defects in his physical condition must be uncovered and dealt with.

In my experience with high school, college, and professional athletes, I have found a condition which does not disable the athlete and may be overlooked; he may be the best player on your team, the best weight lifter you have. He could, however, be better. This condition is called postural imbalance (see figs. 41a, 41b).

This condition exists where one leg is shorter than the other. A tilt of the hips is produced such that the hip on the side of the longer leg is more pronounced or prominent than that on the side of the shorter leg. Usually the spine bends away from the projecting hip at a slightly acute angle, causing tenderness over the sacroiliac joint on the high side, which frequently spreads across the whole lower part of the back. This condition is usually accompanied by a lowering of the shoulder on the side of the longer leg to restore the shoulders to a more horizontal position.

This sometimes produces a semibinding effect on the muscles of the spine. Either leg, more frequently the longer leg, may be affected by numbness on the upper third of the front of the thigh, pain down the side of the leg due to irritation of the sciatic nerve, or occasionally by swelling in one or both legs. However, it should be noted that these symptoms do not always occur as part of the condition.

The effect of this syndrome on an athlete in action is that he will be able to move better to the side of the short leg than to the side of the longer leg. When an athlete, let us say a high-school halfback, favors carrying the ball to the right because he is successful going that way and never moves to the left because he does not seem to move well in that direction, he is impeded by this condition. When he attempts to move to the left (in this case the side of the longer leg) the binding effect inhibits his ability to step off on the left leg; thus he will get only a *stomping half-stride,* thus giving the defense an added split second to move in on him. Moving in the other direction, however, is a different story. The postural imbalance causes the pelvis to be tilted downward and rotated posterially on the side of the shorter leg, rotating the leg and pointing the foot outward from the center of the body, thus offering an advantage to stepping off in this direction. An observant opponent coach might become cognizant of the player's ability to move better in one direction, though he may not really know why this is so.

In weight lifting when one is doing the *clean and jerk,* the *clean* portion of the lift is when the lifter raises the weight from the floor to his shoulder in one motion; he moves under the weight so that it is secured on his shoulders or chest. The *jerk* portion is where the lifter raises the weight from his shoulders to overhead in motion while splitting his legs. The problem arises, for the athlete with a postural imbalance, when he finds that the weight is not level, that the bar is not horizontal, and is lower on the side of the short leg. Feeling this imbalance, he tries to stabilize the weight by raising the right leg to push upward and, in so doing, may injure his elbow, or by twisting the weight to acquire balance, he might fray some of the fibers of the tendons in the anterior side of the wrist area.

Once the imbalance is discovered, osteopathic corrective adjustment removes the tension from the area so that the individual can stand erect. Both the lumbar and sacroiliac areas are relieved. A lift is placed in the shoe of the shorter leg to restore the balance. The patient wears this corrective shoe at all times and never walks in his bare feet. The soreness and stiffness in his back should diminish. Physical therapy and corrective exercises are given and are of great value. After a period of two weeks the individual is brought back, and an x-ray is taken while he's standing in his shoes, and the lift is corrected until there is perfect balance of the pelvis. Following the mechanical correction and the lift placed in the shoe, it is standard policy to practice corrective exercises and physical therapy with these individuals.

For the first exercise the athlete lies flat on his back: then, pulling up his legs with a bend in his knees, he makes a bridge, raising his buttocks into the air; thus the weight will be on his shoulders; he should push up on the count of one, higher on two and drop back to the rest position on three (see figs. 42a, 42b, and 42c). This exercise should be done 10 times a day. This exercise is excellent for lower-back pain, strengthening the back and abdominal muscles, reducing pot belly, and relieves pressure from the lumbar nerves and eliminates slipped or ruptured disc-like symptoms.

After this exercise the patient is then taken to physical therapy. The area where his pain is most severe or most tender is iced down. He is then given ultrasonic treatment over this area for a period of ten minutes, depending on his tolerance.

Assuming that the troubled area involves his right sacroiliac, the patient lies facedown and four Medco-sonolator pads are placed: one

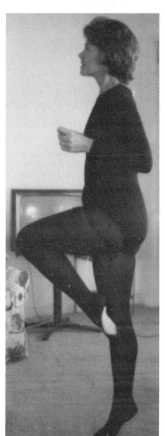

Fig. 23.   Running in place

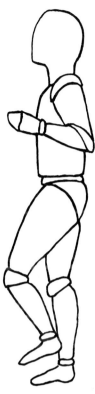

Fig. 24.   10-hop. The form is the same as if running in place except that the knee does not have to be raised as high

Fig. 25.   Ventilation and circulation exercise

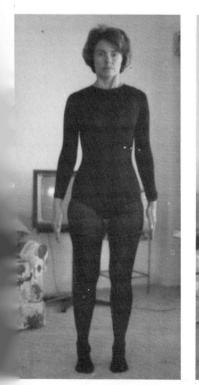

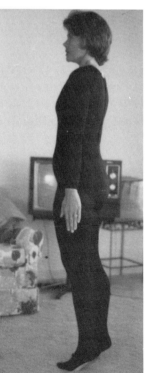

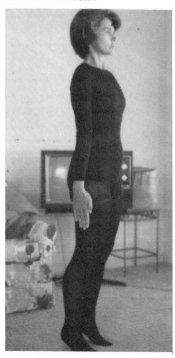

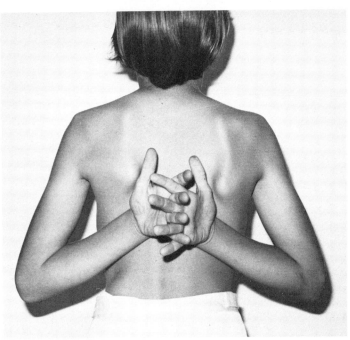

Fig. 26a.   Thumbs up . . .

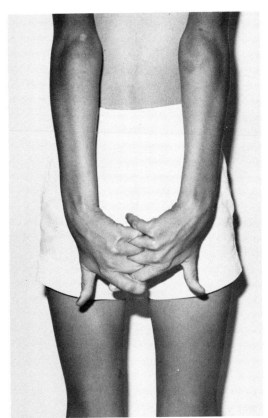

Fig. 26b.   . . . turned . . .

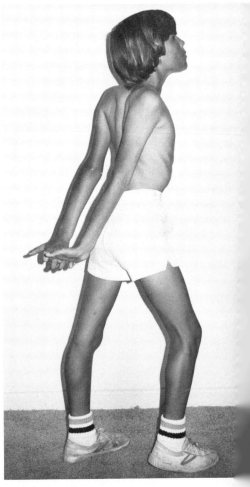

Fig. 26c. . . . palms down

Fig. 28.   The tug-of-war

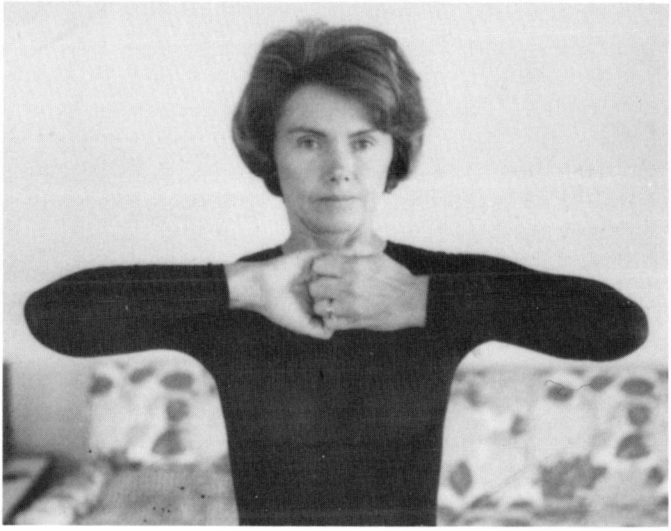

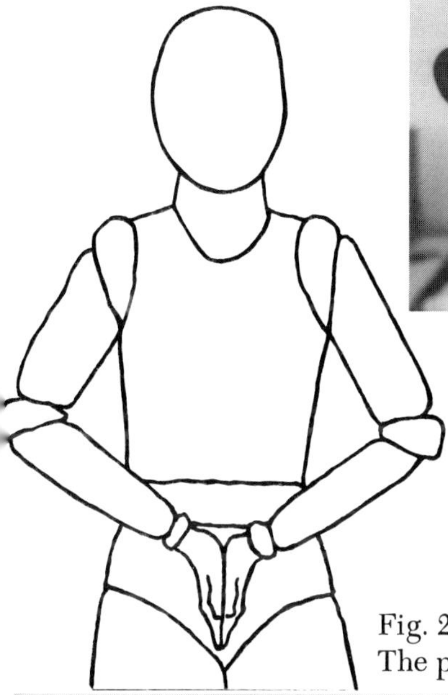

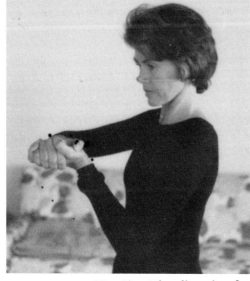

Fig. 27.
The press

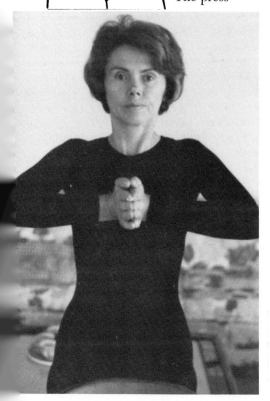

Fig. 29.   The elbow bender

Fig. 30.　The pull

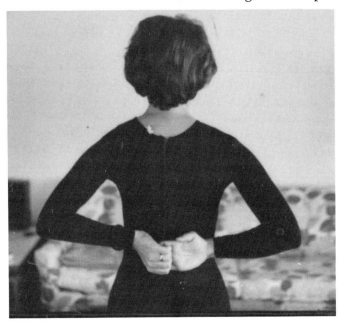

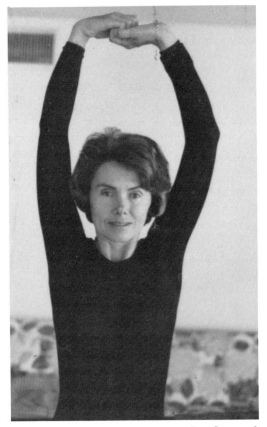

Fig. 32.　Upper-back exercise

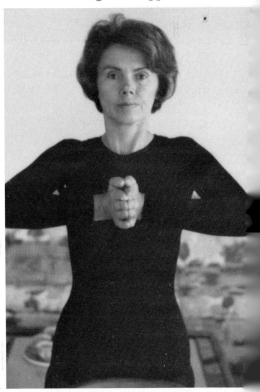

Fig. 31.　Overhead stretch

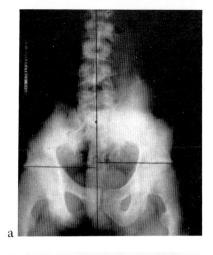

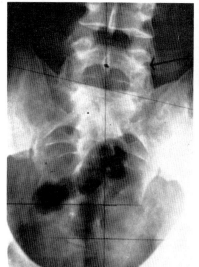

b   Figs. 41a, 41b.   Postural
imbalance

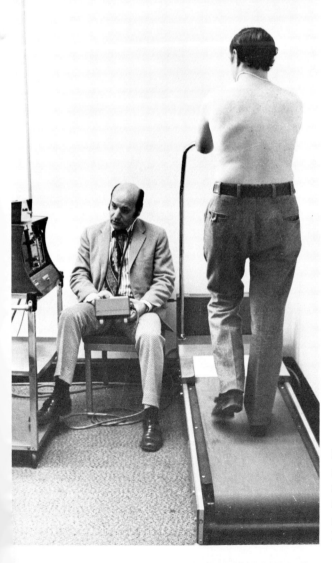

Fig. 34.   The treadmill test is
one of the methods of cardiac
evaluation used in the Cardiac
Consultation Clinic at St. Fran-
cis Hospital and Heart Center,
Roslyn, Long Island, New York

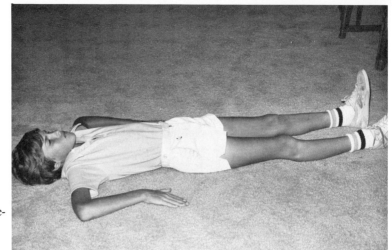

Fig. 42a. Corrective back exercise . . .

Fig. 42b. . . . bridge . . .

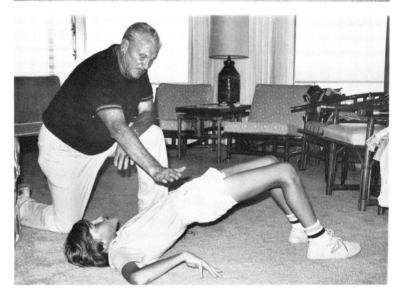

42c. . . . extend and hold

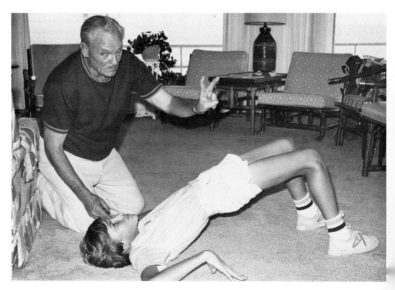

Fig. 46. Wright arch exercisor (depression in right arch indicates placement of spur)

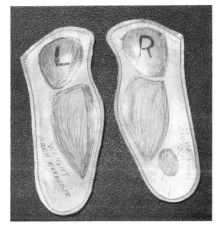

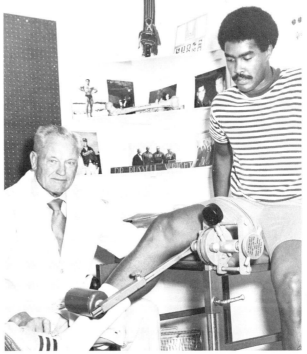

Fig. 48. Developing the quadriceps muscle

Fig. 49. Developing the flexors and rehabilitation of the knee on hydraulic knee exerciser

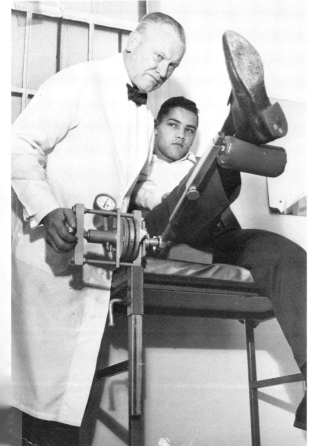

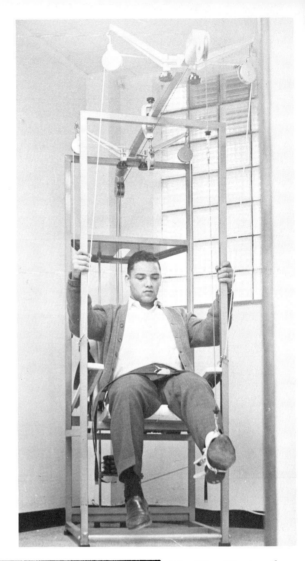

Fig. 50. Developing the extensors and flexors and rehabilitation of knee on Elgin chair

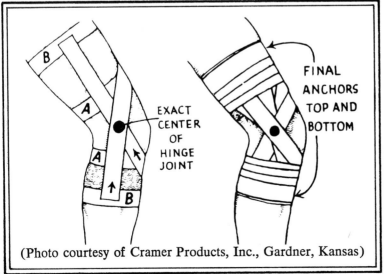

Fig. 51. Taping the knee: *A* and *B* are anchors; vertical strips must cross over at exact center of knee joint. As each pair of vertical strips is applied, anchor above and below. Completed job consists of 8 vertical strips and 4 anchors above and 4 below.

B

A

A

B

EXACT
CENTER
OF
HINGE
JOINT

FINAL
ANCHORS
TOP AND
BOTTOM

(Photo courtesy of Cramer Products, Inc., Gardner, Kansas)

over the left sacroiliac, one over the right, one over the right lumbar area, and one over the right sacrosciatic notch.

A large hydrocolator pack is placed over the area, and the patient is given electrical stimulation for a period of 15 minutes, using a surging type of current to establish better circulation in the area.

His treatment in physical therapy is followed by a trip to the gymnasium, where he is put to work on a power weight rack. He lies down underneath it; weights are placed on the power rack, and he lifts them with his feet, at first pushing them up only a short distance; as he progresses he pushes them all the way up onto his shoulders. It is wise to begin with approximately 100 lbs. on healthy, strong athletes, and then increase the weight up to 300 or 350 lbs. Begin with about 10 reps at first, and if he tires, let him rest. Within a period of 6 weeks, he should be doing about 100 reps at 300 or 350 lbs.

If pain occurs in the patient's leg, it is wise for him to work on a leg-press machine, where he presses up to 50 or 60 lbs. by extending his quadriceps and then pulling back to get his flexors doing the same amount of work so that he can develop the muscles in both the front and back of the thigh.

FEET AND ANKLES

It is important that feet and ankles be as healthy as possible for maximum performance in weight training and weight lifting (see fig. 43). First, let us discuss the heel. A large tendon, the Achilles tendon, runs down the back of the leg and is attached approximately an inch forward

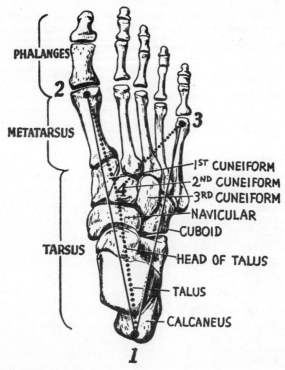

Fig. 43. Anatomy of the Foot (photo courtesy of Cramer Products, Inc., Gardner, Kansas)

from the back of the heel. It is attached to a bony projection, and when this area becomes painful or bruised or a calcium deposit has formed, a spur protrudes from the heel. Spurs have been a problem to athletes for centuries, and many good athletes have been forced to withdraw from competition because of them.

71

What can be done about spurs? What causes them? I've seen cases where spurs practically disappeared of their own accord and just as mysteriously returned. There may be a reason for their appearance. As we walk, the relationship of the heel with other bones of the foot may not be correct, and this relationship creates an abnormal pull on this area. As this abnormal pull comes down from the Achilles tendon, it has a tendency to divert the foot in one direction or the other, depending upon the mechanical malrelation of the arch. Should one happen to get a bruise or burn in the interim, the area becomes sore, the tendon is irritated, calcium may develop, and then the spur forms (see fig. 44). The best treatment for spurs, after they are quieted down, is the manipulation of the foot. While the spur is active, it is well to make a heel pad in the shoe. I prefer to use felt for the pad, possibly something near 3/16 of an inch thick. It may have thin, flexible leather padding over it. Cut a hole in the back center area about 1 inch from where the heel bone would be; then have the patient fit them into his shoes and try them. Many people to whom I have recommended this treatment said they were much worse, and it was true. This was because the hole in the heel pad was not cut far enough forward, and the sharp edges of the spur or the anatomical prominence where the Achilles tendon attaches hits the edge of that heel pad, which, in turn, would make it worse as the spur is not centered into the pad to relieve the irritation. This treatment has relieved the pain and congestion in most cases; the foot is restored to its normal relationship and usually the pain and soreness disappear.

In our discussion of the foot, we move on to the arch, also known as a transverse arch or crossways, composed of seven bones. While

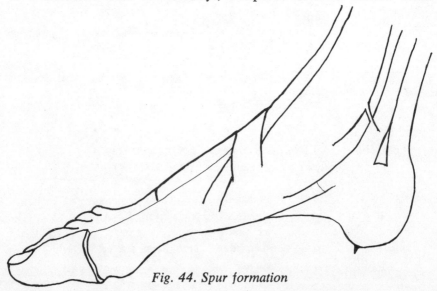

Fig. 44. Spur formation

playing baseball, a right-handed batter might foul a ball off the arch of his foot, or in weight lifting or weight training the lifter may drop a weight which might hit the arch of his foot. As it hits the arch, the object drives it down; as it comes back up, the bones may not rise in their normal relationship. The person might try to run, but the bones will not move. He has to drag this one foot because it is too painful to lift. Usually its the medial cuneiform, or the bone that lies nearer the inside of the foot, that doesn't reach its normal position. This, in turn, affects that whole transverse arch and makes it impossible for a person to run; the area is tender. There is a manner of manipulation which can correct and restore the foot's normal physiological motion.

The next area of the foot as we approach the toes is what we call the longitudinal arch, composed of five metacarpal bones. What can happen to this area? One condition common during wartime was march fracture. During long marches, the foot became so fatigued that, as it dropped down, one of the bones in the longitudinal arch developed a hairline fracture, as opposed to a displacing fracture, missed most of the time in x-rays. This patient had a very painful foot, especially when walking any distances. When this condition is determined, the treatment, of course, is removing pressure from it; the foot usually makes an uneventful recovery (see fig. 45 for taping instructions).

Next we arrive at the toes. In each toe there are three bones, except for the large or big toe; it has two. What can happen to the toes? An infection or fungus might appear under the toenails. It will appear as a powdery substance. This should be well cleaned out and the toenails kept clean.

The big toe may develop an ingrown toenail. There is no reason for this to happen. The nail of the large toe should be cut square across. The midline of that toenail can be straight or filed down so that it is not thick and then a wedge shape cut in the toenail so that the outside of the toenail will extend out over the flesh of the toe; instead of being turned down and cutting into the skin, the nail will extend and grow out over the edge of the toe. This is the effect you want. If the toenail grows out past the soft tissue of the toe, and the corners are out beyond, then they will not be digging into the tissues to cause an ingrown toenail, which might become infected and very painful. Should this happen, and the nail be grown deep into the skin, after the infection is cleared up, remove about ¼ to ⅓ of that toenail on the side of the affected area well back into the nail bed, and as a wedge of tissue is removed from the soft tissue below the nail, then it can be approximated and the excess tissue removed and turned down. Then, as the toenail grows it will grow out over the tissue and not into it, thus eliminating the ingrown toenail.

Another problem which might develop is known as a plantar's wart;

Fig. 45. Taping the Longitudinal Arch (photo and text courtesy of
Cramer Products, Inc., Gardner, Kansas)

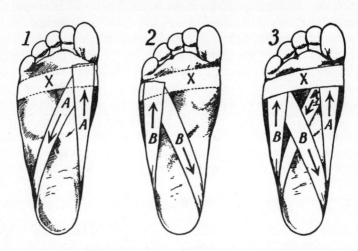

This is the unofficially approved method of taping for
a sprained longitudinal arch of the foot. Some coaches use
this method for shin splint.

1. Apply Q.D.A. or Tuf-Skin.

2. Apply an anchor around the foot as outlined by area
"X" dotted lines. This anchor should not be snug, as the
arch will increase in width when standing.

3. Start the tape at "A", cross the foot, go around the
heel and back up to "A".

4. The second strip "B" is similar to "A" but on the opposite side of the foot.

5. Apply another anchor at "X" over the tape ends of
both "A" and "B". Again carry the anchor around the foot.

These strips "A" and "B" must not be applied with great
pressure. Remember, the foot is normally about ½" longer
when it carries the weight of the body.

Note particularly the position of the strips "A" and "B"
under the first and fifth toes. This position should be maintained.

many boys and girls have these warts, which can be treated in the following manner. First, of course, consult your physician; for temporary relief of the pressure, however, cut a circle out of felt and cut a hole in the center. If the wart is ¼ inch in diameter, the hole should be ½ inch in diameter. Place it so that the wart is inside the ring; then put a Band-Aid or a piece of tape over it so that pressure forms around it, not on it. There are other methods of treating these warts—x-ray therapy, carbon dioxide, acids—and some of them end the problem. Sometimes, however, there is no other way to treat them except by surgery.

If an irritation or cracking between the toes develops, and there is evidence of a fungus infection, there are powder products that can be sprayed there to give relief and take care of the burning and itching that go along with this condition.

Between the fourth and fifth toes, the small and little toe, a bending of that little toe and pressure in the area may cause a callus to form, well known as a corn. It's a deposit of tissue that forms to stop the sharp edge of bone of the joint that is hitting into the other toe. To remove the pressure from this, place a little cotton in between those toes to act as a pad. If the corn is large, crush an aspirin tablet, moisten it, and lay it in between the toe and over the area; bandage it with tape. The next morning it will have dehydrated the callus enough so that it can be lifted from the toe without any bleeding or irritation.

There is much discussion on the subject of flat feet. Many people have been told their feet are flat, when in reality they are not. How can you tell? If you get out of a pool and walk and you can see the imprint of your toes, your heel and the ball of your foot, but no mark is left to indicate the inside of your arch, then you don't have flat feet; you have an arch that is fairly well up in its position. If, however, you see almost a flat foot mark when you get out of a pool, then you have flat feet. Flat feet can be tiring, and treatments include types of splints, braces, and arch supports. I prefer to use the *Wright* exercisor (see fig. 46), which I designed and have used for 45 years.

It is important that the section of the shoes under the transverse arch be built up, usually with leather, wool, and possibly rubber so that there's not a hard resilience but a pumping and springing effect with some pressure. It is important not to lose the effect of this spring in your foot. A solid metal arch does not allow for such spring. It would be like riding in a wagon without springs or shock absorbers.

Sometimes a metatarsal block is set a half inch behind the heads of metatarsal articulation or their junction. The block should be the correct length and width so that it conforms to the foot. Then the arch is supported; the patient gets a pumping and springing effect. He will have comfort and won't get that tiredness and low backache and pressure down through his legs.

It's been said that you get over every sprained ankle you've ever had except the first one, and I think that's true, unless it is corrected by mechanical manipulation, restoring all metatarsal bones to their right relationships with each other and their neighbors. When one sprains his ankle and frays or stretches some of the ligaments, the ankle turns from the outside; in other words, the ankle is turned over and the injury occurs. What happens later is that the individual steps on a rough spot, rolling gravel, or uneven ground, and the ankle tips over and throws him since the foot is facing in toward the midline instead of being flat on the floor. When this condition exists, one must look (as with the case of a spur) for a mechanical malrelation in one of the bones of the ankle; this is usually indicated by tenderness on palpation. When this is determined, the condition can usually be corrected by mechanical manipulation (see fig. 47 for the Louisiana Wrap).

Fig. 47. The Louisiana Wrap (photo and text courtesy of
Cramer Products, Inc., Gardner, Kansas)

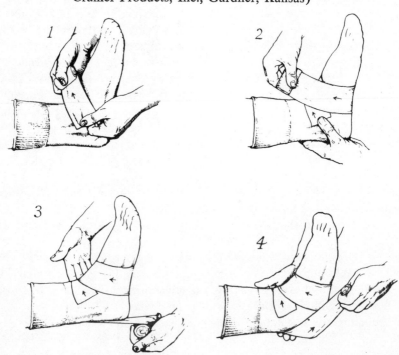

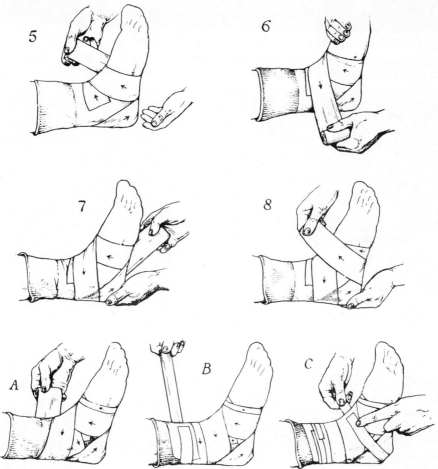

You have completed a single lift on each side of the heel. For 72″ wrap—spiral up the ankle and secure as shown in A, B and C.

For a 96″ wrap—repeat steps 3 to 8 inclusive, for 2 heel "lifts" and spiral up ankle.

The wrap is spiraled up over the ankle as shown in A, B and C. Two pieces of tape are used to secure, one around the top (B) and one across the heel (C). For the completed job a 96″ wrap is used. It would be wise to practice this method until application is perfected and correct pressure is obtained.

WHEN APPLIED OVER A SOCK, USE FIRM PRESSURE.

Remember, spurs and sprained ankles are due primarily to an abnormal pull on the tendons in the foot due to a mechanical malrelation of the bones in the arch of the foot.

KNEES AND MORE KNEES

I have been examining and treating weight lifters for the past seventeen years, and over 50 percent of their complaints concern their knees. In fact, the first weight lifter I examined and treated had a knee problem, and he had been sent to my Detroit office. Would he still be able to lift in spite of his knee condition? I immediately examined the knee for any unusual injuries; it was also x-rayed on several planes, but the x-rays were negative. When I examined the knee more thoroughly, the individual experienced considerable pain inside the front of the knee below the cap. He also had pain when the kneecap was pushed right and left, and especially when pressure was placed on the interior pole of the kneecap and it was shoved forward or pressure placed on the back of the kneecap. The maximum pain, however, seemed to be inside the knee below the cap, and the lifter had pain if he did a deep squat carrying no weight and having his buttocks hit his heels. When I put him on a leg-extension machine, and he tried to stretch 30 or 40 lbs. to a 180° level, he had severe pain when relieved from extension pressure; when he pulled back wide open to the extreme end of the flexors, he had more pain. (Figures 48 through 50 demonstrate basic knee exercises for rehabilitating knees after injury or surgery.)

It was determined that there were adhesions underneath the patella. The knee was injected with an anesthetic and then manipulatd to free these adhesions. The knee was injected in the lower right quadrant on the edge of the kneecap with a 26-gauge, 1½-inch needle, also injecting the opposite side at the time.

It is very difficult to inject the anesthetic from the right side into the left, directing the injection on both sides of the midline underneath the kneecap, while at the same time being careful to inject between the membranes, not into them, and to place the solution in an open area space.

This condition may also occur at the superior part of the kneecap or along the edges of either lateral or medial side. Wherever they are present, they must be freed and the kneecap extended and allowed to go through its normal range of motion when the man is in a deep bend position. Usually a steroid or cortisone is mixed with the xylocain and injected into this area. However, long before steroids, novocaine was injected. So cortisone is a newcomer as far as treatment for this condition is concerned.

I'm of the opinion, after many years of study, that the greatest cause for this knee problem in weight lifters is their taking too much weight too soon and not warming up. They want to go into the gym and immediately do a deep squat with heavy weights instead of warming up adequately and building up strength.

I have, on occasion, found many lifters with patella irritation. After they received the anesthetic injection, I put this knee through its normal range of motion physically by extending it and taking the kneecap in my hand as if it were a plane, pushing it forward, backward, sideways and around to separate all of the adhering structures so that the kneecap will go through its full, normal range of motion when the lifter moves into the squat position. Following the manipulation, he is then taken to the gym where he will use a weight-press machine, extending his leg out to 180°, pulling his leg back as far as he can underneath to an acute angle (about 60°) and through this range of motion, lifting all that he can, anywhere from 30 to 80 lbs. Freeing any other areas under the knee with the pressure, he will not defend the knee and will be able to move it freely because of the anesthetic.

After this workout, the individual uses a power lift, raising 100 to 150 lbs. of weight or up to 50 kilos, doing several repetitions up to a dozen. Then he is taken to physical therapy, where he receives electrical stimulation under a hydrocolator pack, to establish good drainage and stimulation throughout the area. The patient is then discharged and returns daily for treatment for one full week following this, doing squats and buttock bounces to determine if there are any further adhesions in need of correction. If he is free of pain and adhesions, he is able to resume his lifting program.

In summation, it is my belief that weight lifters have knee problems because they do not warm up properly; they take too much weight too fast. My advice to all young weight lifters is to do your deep squat at first slowly and with a broom handle, doing more repetitions, just going through the motions; then gradually add a little more weight, and take a considerable time before you put pressure on the leg. Build up all the strength you need before you throw into the heavy weight (see fig. 51 for instruction on knee taping).

OSTEOPATHIC
MANIPULATIVE THERAPY

Osteopathic manipulative therapy is utilized to restore the normal physiological motion to the disarranged segments of the musculoskeletal system. There are two methods of therapy.

1. Direct therapy applies force to the restrictor of motion of the involved segment or area.

2. Indirect therapy reflects the force away from the restrictor of motion toward the area of mobility and attempts to restore normalcy of function.

Force may be applied by the physician by means of gravity, physical traction, or intrinsic force generated by the patient (including respiratory contraction, muscular contraction, isometric or isotonic contraction) or the inherent energy forces of the body. Combined therapies (direct and indirect) can use intrinsic or extrinsic force. Osteopathic manipulative therapy must be individualized for each patient as accurately as any other medical treatment.

I've found that osteopathic corrective adjustment, postural balance, and corrective exercises, along with supportive treatments (including electrical stimulation, ultrasonic treatment, whirlpool baths, hot and cold packs) and rhythmic traction to the affected area have put athletes back into the games and transformed an ordinary athlete into a star.

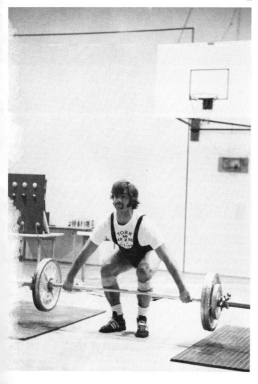
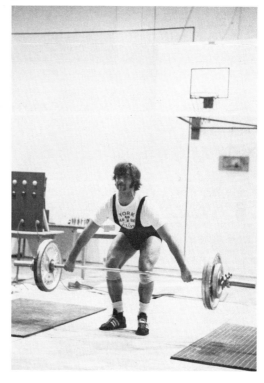

a b

Figs. 52a-52g. From snatch to squat *(Photos of Mark Cameron courtesy of Bruce Klemens)*

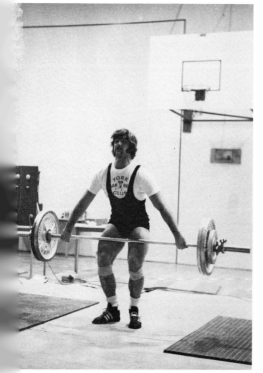

c

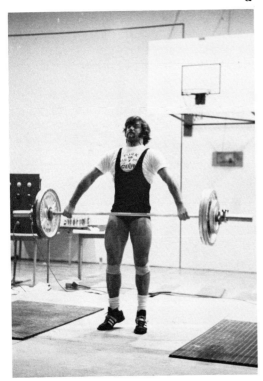 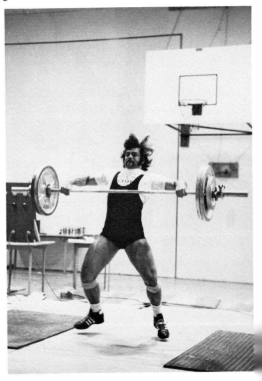

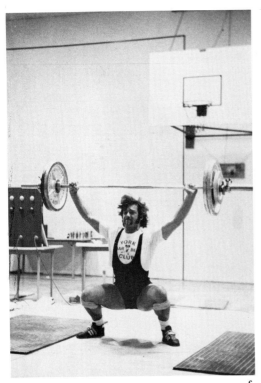 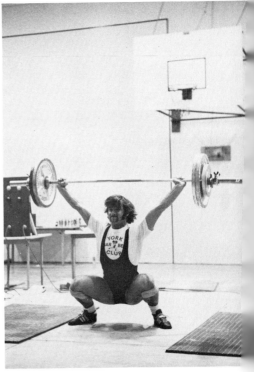

a

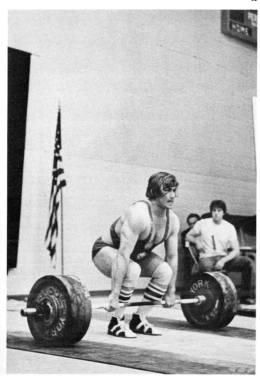

Figs. 53a-53p. The clean and jerk
*(Photos of Ernie Petersen courtesy
of Bruce Klemens)*

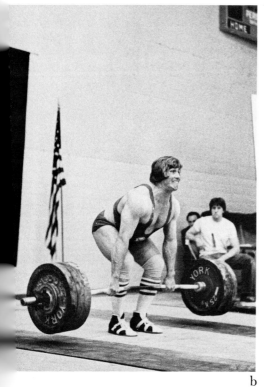

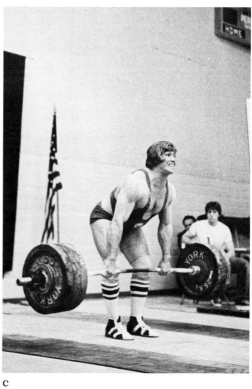

b   c

d e

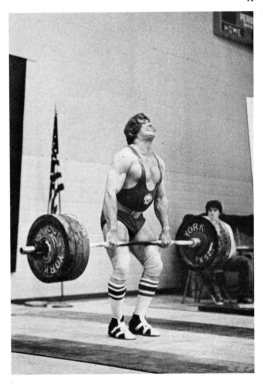 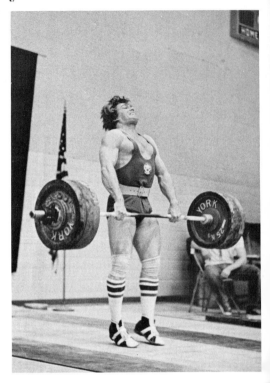

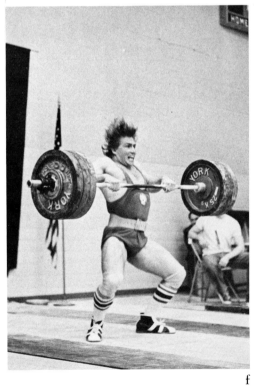 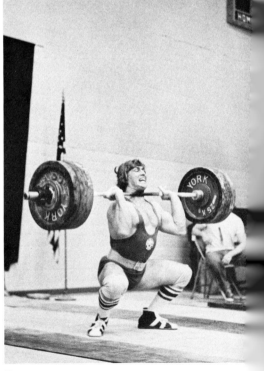

f g

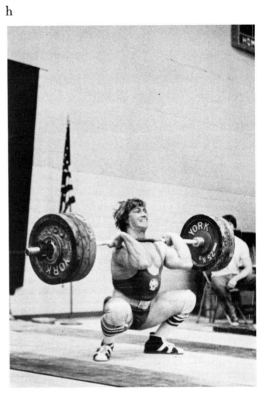

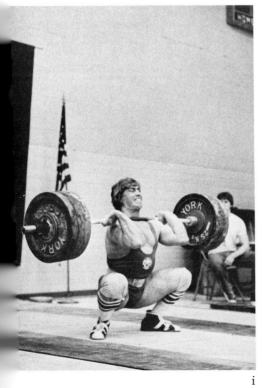

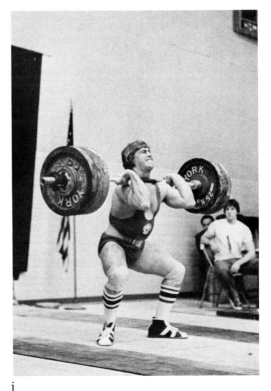

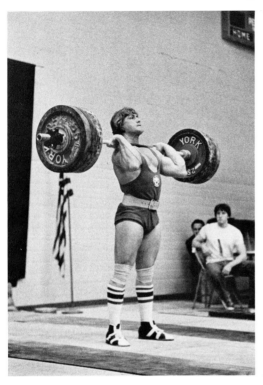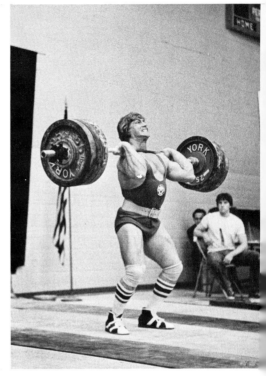

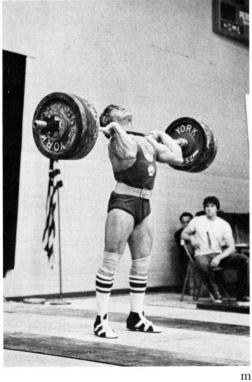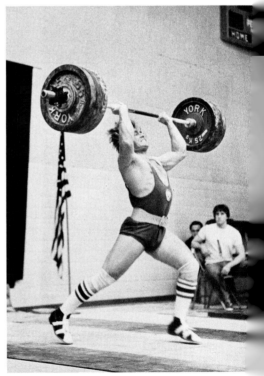

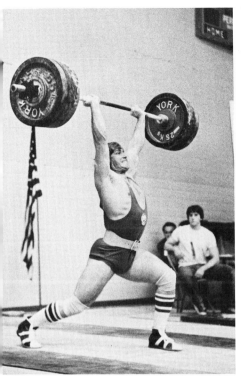
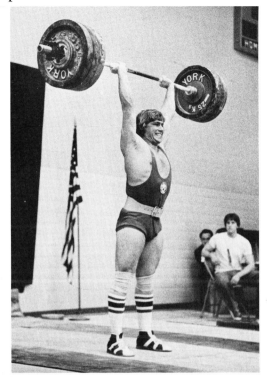
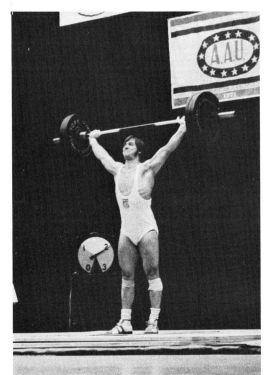

Fig. 54. Completed snatch *(Photo of Rick Holbrook courtesy of Bruce Klemens)*

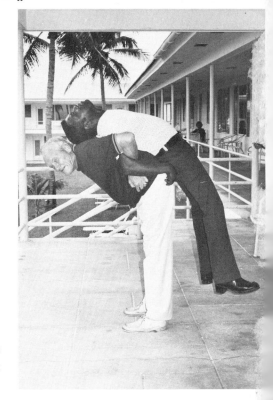

Figs. 55a, 55b, 55c. Corrective treatment for acute spasm in back muscles and sacroiliac strain

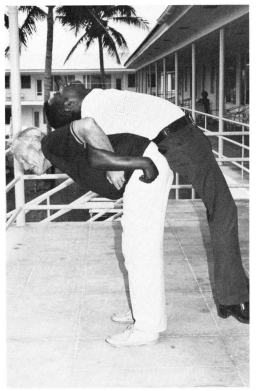

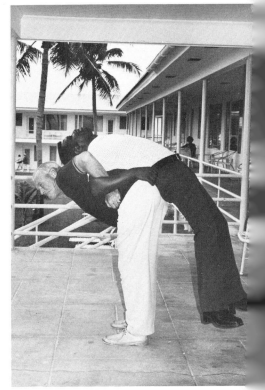

b   c

WEIGHT-LIFTING TECHNIQUES

WEIGHT-LIFTING TECHNIQUES

The lifting of heavy weights is practiced by millions of athletes in junior high schools, high schools, colleges, semipro and professional sports. However, if one is training for weight lifting as a sport to participate in the local association, regional, national, international or Olympic meetings, there are definite rules of procedure as well as lifts to be performed. Two of these lifts are the *two-hand snatch* (see figs. 52a through 52g) and the *clean and jerk* (see figs. 53a through 53p).

It has been stated that the snatch is the fastest of any single movement in the entire Olympic games. The snatch is when the lifter raises the weight from the floor to overhead in one motion. It usually involves the lifter pulling the weight to at least the lower-chest height and, before the weight starts to come back down, quickly pulling his body under the weight so that it is secured overhead and held on straight arms. The lifter then quickly pushes his legs up to an erect position. An experienced weight lifter can perform this complete sequence with rapid speed.

There are two styles commonly used to go under the weight. First is the *squat* style. Here the lifter pulls his body under the weight while moving his legs to the side in a squat or a deep-knee-bend position. The second is known as the *split* style. Here the lifter pulls his body under the weight while moving one of his legs forward in a bent position and the other leg back in a straight position. In both styles, the lifter recovers to the erect position while keeping the weight at arm's length.

The Snatch. Place your feet close to the weight or the bar; your feet should be about a shoulder width apart. Stand erect with a slight arch in your back. Bending your legs, reach down and grasp the weight at a width wider than your shoulder. Lift the weight by straightening your legs and extending your body until you are fully upright. Then squat or split under the weight. It is very important to keep the weight close to your body during the pull and to fully extend your legs and shoulders upward. The finish of the pull should have the lifter on his toes with his shoulders shrugged upward. The weight should be pulled upward, rather than backward or forward. It's very important that this weight goes in a direct track, being elevated upward and not backward or forward. After you stand upright, holding the weight at arm's length under control, the referee should give you the nod. Then you can place it back on the platform, which is the end of a perfect lift (fig. 54 shows a completed snatch). It takes speed, training, coordination, flexibility, motivation, and determination to make a good snatch lift.

The Clean and Jerk. The clean and jerk is commonly referred to as the king of lifts. The reason for this is that the clean and jerk is where the most weight can be lifted overhead from the floor. The portion of the lift known as the clean is when the lifter raises the weight from the floor to the shoulders in one motion. The lifter raises the weight at least waist height and, before the weight start coming back down, pulls his body under the weight so that he has it secured on his shoulders or chest. The lifter then stands erect. The jerk is where the lifter raises the weight just cleaned from his shoulders overhead in one motion while splitting his legs. The lifter then stands erect. Unlike the snatch, when the lifter pulls himself underneath the weight for the clean, the weight ends up at his shoulders, not overhead. The elbows end up forward of the weight. Recovery to straight legs from the squat or split completes the clean.

To start the clean, place your feet close to the weight (feet should be shoulder width or less apart), and stand erect with a slight arch in your back and your legs. Reach down and grasp the weight with a shoulder-width grip. Lift the weight by straightening your legs and extending your body until you are fully upright. At this time you squat or split under the weight. It is very important to keep the weight close to your body during the pull and to fully extend your legs and shoulders upward. The finish of the pull should have the lifter on his toes with his shoulders shrugged upward. The weight should be pulled upward, rather than backward or forward. Most of the fouls or loss of weight occur when the bar is too far forward or backward and you lose that straight line. After you stand upright with the weight at your shoulders, you are ready to jerk the weight.

To perform the jerk, bend your legs so that the weight is 4 to 8 inches below the finished clean position. Maintain your torso in the upright position during this time and during the complete jerk. Immediately straighten your legs, thereby accelerating the weight upward. As your legs straighten, continue pushing the weight off your torso by using your shoulders and arms. As the weight approaches its high point, split your legs, pushing up strongly on the weight to maintain weight at arm's length. Now straighten your legs or shove them up so that you are completely upright with the weight firmly at arm's length. This completes the jerk. It is important not to allow the weight to sag on your torso or to let the torso bend forward during the jerk. The weight should be held high on the torso. The weight should be driven upward, not forward or backward. After you stand upright with the weight at arm's length, you are then ready for the signal from the referee to place the weight back on the platform.

WEIGHT TRAINING

WEIGHT TRAINING

For each exercise select a weight you can lift six times without strain. When you have progressed to the point where you can lift the weight 10 times without strain, add 5 pounds. In each exercise do three sets of 6 to 10 repetitions. Rest after completing each set.

For the Arms

1. CURLS

Starting position: Stand erect, feet shoulder-width apart. Hold bar down in front of body, with palms facing *outward* and shoulder-width apart. *Action:* Count 1 —Curl the bar upward to the chin, bending arms at elbows. Count 2—Return to starting position.

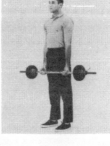 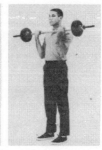

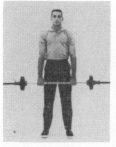 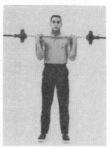

2. REVERSE CURLS

Starting position: Stand erect, feet shoulder-width apart. Hold bar down in front of body, with palms facing *inward* and shoulder-width apart. *Action:* Count 1— Curl the bar upward to the chin, bending arms at elbows. Count 2—Return to starting position.

3. STANDING PRESS

Starting position: Stand erect, supporting weight at shoulder level, with feet and hands shoulder-width apart. *Action:* Count 1—Press weight overhead to extended-arm position. Count 2—Return to starting position.

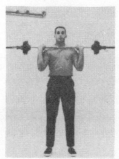 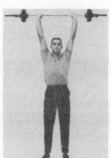

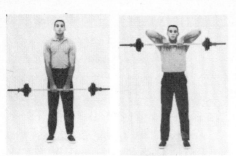

For the Shoulders
1. PULLUPS
Starting position: Stand erect, feet shoulder-width apart. Hold bar down in front of body, with palms facing inward and 2 to 3 inches apart. *Action:* Count 1—Pull bar up to chin, holding elbows high. Count 2—Return to starting position.

For the Chest
1. PRONE PRESS
Starting position: Lie on back on floor or bench, with legs straight. Support weight with palms facing out and spaced shoulder-width apart. *Action:* Count 1—Press weight up to extended-arm position. Count 2—Return slowly to starting position.

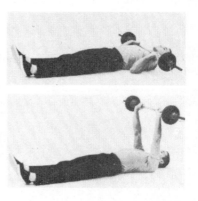

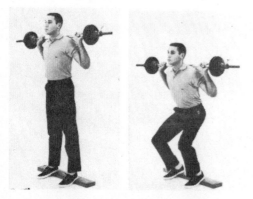

For the Legs
1. HALF SQUATS
Starting position: Stand erect, feet shoulder-width apart, with weight supported across shoulders. *Action:* Count 1—Bend knees halfway. Count 2—Return to starting position. A support under the heels will improve balance.

Section V

DRUGS AND THE WEIGHT LIFTER

DOPING

Doping is the administration to the use by a healthy individual while taking part in a sporting competition of:

A. Any chemical agent or substance not normally present in the body and which does not play either an essential or normal part in the day-to-day biochemical environment or processes of metabolism regardless of the dosage, preparation or route of administration and/or

B. Any chemical agent or substance which plays an essential or normal part in the day-to-day process of metabolism or performs a normal part of the biochemical environment when introduced in abnormal quantities and/or by an abnormal route or in abnormal form. Either or both of which are present in the body of an individual during competition for the purpose or with the effect of modifying artificially the performance of the individual during competition.

The following drug substances must never be used for the treatment of sportsmen and sportswomen while they are actually taking part in sports competitions:

1. Alcohol, specifically ethyl alcohol.
2. Amphetamines and their derivatives.
3. Purion bases, camphor and pharmacodynamically including the amaleptics, cocaine, diglan and similar substances.
4. Monoamine oxidase inhibitors, Lobelline and similar substances.
5. Nitrates and similar substances.
6. Peripheral vasodilators; Phenothiazines; strychnine; Picrotoxin, Tropeines; narcotics; Uridine triphosphate.
7. Hormones (including those of the corticosteroid and applied series) when given systemically unless they have been regularly used by the patients for a period of 28 days.

The use of steroids for suppression of menstrual periods in female competitors may be taken to be excluded from this ban pending further classification and international discussion.

The use of anabolic steroids is considered unethical and should be on the forbidden list.

At an Olympic meeting or a world championship the rules of the International Olympic Committee are followed. The drugs tested for are

95

usually done from urine specimens. When a world championship is taking place, there are usually three award winners; a gold, silver and bronze winner. These three are tested along with two other sportsmen picked at random. These two random individuals are picked from secret numbers, and they are picked by the physician representing the I.W.F. in charge that day. These numbers are not known until the end of the competition when the individuals are called and the individual having the number that has been selected is also called for examination. Should there be two sessions in the Olympics, an afternoon and evening session, the three winners in the afternoon session are selected and tested. This would make a total of eight people being chosen and examined for drugs on that particular day. As soon as the competition has been completed, the individuals to be tested go to the first-aid or to the drug-testing room. The sportsman is accompanied by his coach, trainer or physician. There he is given a sterile beaker and under the direct view of the I.W.F. examining physician on duty, the sportsman will produce a specimen of from 4 to 6 ounces of urine in the beaker. This specimen is divided into two bottles; each bottle has a mark placed on it, a number which is secret and which the competitor has selected. It will be cut in each glass; his name, country and coach are recorded. One jar goes to the laboratory, and the second jar is closed with wax and a seal stamped on it. The second specimen is placed in a refrigerator under lock and key, the physician on duty being the only one who has a key to this refrigerator. This specimen is then labeled so that no one knows the name of the specimen, only the number and that number is only known by the physician on duty and the athlete and his coach. If a positive reaction is found on the first specimen, the athlete is called in before the drug committee. At this meeting he can admit his guilt or request the second specimen be tested in case of error.

ANABOLIC STEROIDS

It was a great pleasure and honor for the author to be selected as a delegate to both the F.I.M.S. and the Technical Commission Meeting in London in 1975.

Many of the great men in sport representing problems of athletes, universities and research were present to deliver papers or comment on the subject. Naming them all would require entirely too much space. The officers of the F.I.M.S. (Federation International Medicine Sportive) were present. Dr. La Cava, Dr. Prokop, Dr. Plas, Dr. Dirix, Dr. Williams and two well-known sportsmen, Dr. Arne Ljungquist and Dr. Roger Bannister, as well as many, many more. The results of this meeting were published in volume 9, number 2 of the *British Journal of Sports Medicine.*

Following are the conclusions of the F.I.M.S. at the end of the meeting:

1. The actions of anabolic steroids in healthy, training athletes are not fully understood. Studies show conflicting results in respect to increase in body size, measures of strength and improvement in performance. The use of anabolic steroids appears, however, to be widespread in certain sports. The difficulties of trial procedures are noted, especially in respect to ethical consideration.

2. Biological studies demonstrate side effects of anabolic steroids such as gonadal and pituitary suppression and hepatic and prostatic involvement; in addition psychological effects should be considered. The muscle bulk increased due to anabolics is due mainly to water retention.

3. Detection methods for anabolic steroids, as well as naturally occurring hormones, are effective, and we seek a wider spread of approved testing laboratories to eliminate the use of the drugs in sports.

The following day, the F.I.M.S. Technical Commission Meeting concluded:

1. This meeting considering the evidence of the London symposium (19.2.75) and previous evidence condemns the prescription of anabolic steroids by physicians for healthy persons participating in sports.

2. This meeting recommends the International Federation to implement effective anabolic steroid control methods relevant to each sport throughout the year.

We shall discuss anabolic steroids under five headings:
1. History
2. The effect
3. The use of anabolic steroids in athletes
4. Detection of anabolic steroids, particularly anabol and dianabol
5. The enforcement

Let us list those as A, B, C, D, and E.

Under Number A it is general knowledge that rapid weight gains occur in boys and girls with the onset of puberty and an increase in their growth rate. The physical differences between men and women are fairly well recognized by most people; the more muscular male owes his mainly to the testosterone, and the female curves mainly are due to adipose tissue or to an estrogenic effect. The protein anabolic effect of testosterone is well recognized and can be exploited therapeutically. The term "anabolic" implies that the substance under consideration is being synthesized and stored. In the context of today's discussion, the term "anabolic steroid" refers to compounds which increase the production of protein in the body.

Testosterone is the most powerful of all the anabolic steroids in humans and is already mentioned as responsible for the greater muscle mass of men compared with women.

Anabolic steroids taken orally have shown many unwanted effects and should really be regarded as highly dangerous compounds which should not be used except under careful medical supervision, and even then they have only a restricted use in therapy.

The orally active anabolic steroids are hepato-toxic and cause cholestatic jaundice. Long, continued use may be associated with liver tumors, including cancers. It is, however, the potential atherogenic risk of these compounds that I wish to stress. The accelerated development of the atherosclerosis, which leads to heart disease, stroke and peripheral vascular disease, can be anticipated when drugs cause disturbances in carbohydrates and lipid metabolism.

The orally active anabolic steroids can do this. It has also been reported in the research that they upset the insulin metabolism, and in the diabetic or the prediabetic this might cause considerable difficulty. One can note the interference with glucose tolerance. The glucose tolerance, as you know, determines the amount of sugar in the blood over a period of time to determine whether or not a prediabetic condition exists.

I would like to stress that, in my view, there is no justification for the use of orally active anabolic steroids in healthy subjects. They have a very restricted medical usefulness, and their use requires close medical supervision.

In athletes large dosages of anabolic steroids have reduced the output of testosterone and gonadotropin, and similar effects have been noticed in rats.

It may be, therefore, that anabolic steroids do not exert their effect on muscles which are not simultaneously exercised, a point which could perhaps improve their reputation in the spheres for which they are originally marked—debility and convalescence. Indeed it has been the experience of one of the researchers at this clinic that if a particular muscle group escapes exercise during the training, it fails to show the improvement that the other muscles display. Reports of athletes and men taking anabolic steroids show that there is a lower incidence of training injuries, and, if they do occur, they heal more quickly. There is said to be a general decrease in fatigability, allowing for longer and more strenuous and more frequent training sessions.

Now let's look at the problem from the ethical standpoint. We do not believe that the acquisition of knowledge in itself justifies the performance of an immoral procedure, and we are aware that the taking of anabolic steroids for athletic reasons can be criticized on at least two ethical grounds. First, it may give the competitor an unfair advantage over opponents who are not taking them. Second, it is wrong to give a drug to a healthy person.

Dr. A. Ljungquist of Stockholm, an Olympic athlete and now a fine physician, reported that 75 percent of the athletes using anabolic steroids experienced an increase in body weight. Most of these athletes also experienced an increase in appetite and in muscular mass. Mental disorders slight in nature were reported by a number of athletes. Some of these said that they had become more aggressive and active; others reacted in the opposite manner.

In only a limited number of athletes had blood chemistry examinations been performed, and some of them had an elevation of serum cholesterol, and GOT and GPT were recorded. No jaundice was recorded. It is concluded from this meeting and from the Swedish reports that the use of anabolic steroids appears to be rather widespread among top athletes, particularly throwers and weight lifters.

Any effects on the competition results appear to be very questionable since most of the athletes who improved their results also had a harder training period. In addition, a significant number of athletes who had been using anabolic steroids and training harder had not improved their results. Certain side effects may appear as a consequence of the use of anabolic steroids. The present investigation has only recorded short-term side effects thus far, which have not been of any medical importance.

Dr. A. H. Payne of the University of Birmingham, England, discussed athletes' points of view. How do they themselves feel about the subject? Many British athletes have been questioned in an attempt to discover what their thinking is. I must say, however, that unless one has been a serious athlete himself, it is difficult to understand the internal and external pressures present when faced with the choice. It takes a strong will indeed to go against the very drive and ambition that make one such a competitive athlete.

"Shall I compete at a lower level than other athletes?" asked one member of the team. Think further of the athlete taking steroids. In spite of his guilt feeling, he is overjoyed with the effects at first, but there is a diminishing return when increasing the dose. Then he begins to worry about his opposition being on a stronger dose, or maybe even on a better, improved drug.

Undoubtedly, there are psychological effects resulting from the use of steroids. The ones who benefit most from the effects are the nervous competitors who suddenly find the confidence to lift themselves out of mediocrity. They are the ones who would likely have to come off the drugs if psychological testing is done. The majority of athletes spoken to, however, would welcome the test if they could insure that no drug takers in the world would escape detection. Athletes, as a whole, do not want to take steroids.

Who is to blame for the present confusion about anabolic steroids? Don't pin all the blame on the athletes. The distribution of steroids is controlled by law, and few athletes could obtain them without the help of doctors. This is true in most countries. Coaches have a difficult job to do. On the one hand, their worth is reflected by the performances of the athletes they coach; on the other hand, they bear tremendous responsibility regarding the power and influence they exert over their athletes.

Great strides have been made in steroid detection. Dr. R. V. Brooks and his aides at St. Thomas Hospital in London have discovered that anabolic steroids have special features which distinguish them from natural steroid hormones. Therefore, it would be possible to detect their use by testing either the blood or urine. At present there are three effective techniques to determine their presence. It has been discovered that the effects of anabolic steroids may last 10 days after taking them. The amount discovered in the blood was still very heavily concentrated, and it is believed that positive effects may still be felt up to 30 days or longer after taking the drug.

These tests were developed to be highly accurate, and time was not considered an element. The next phase is to speed up the tests so they can be reported within a reasonable length of time. At present we can have results in 24 hours, and the tests can be simplified to save both time and money. At present there are a number of laboratories worldwide that are able to do these particular tests.

Recent data available lists the results of studies on anabolic steroids. Metabolites have been identified and characterized: also noted are the principal ions which may be used for the specific detection by selection of ion monitoring. Many studies on the metabolic effect of anabolic steroids are still incomplete. It has been shown, however, that most compounds can be detected as metabolites in the urine.

One problem that has been resolved is that steroids now must be identified by name. The I.A.A.F. rules require the actual doping substance to be identified beyond reasonable doubt, and the International Sports Federation has recently requested the I.O.C. to make the holding of any doping control the condition for the grant of the I.O.C. patronage in area games.

If this is enforced, it will greatly assist us in extending fully comprehensive control to all the major international competitions. This extension of control will inevitably increase the need for qualified medical officers to supervise the procedures at our meetings, but I am confident that the help we shall need will be forthcoming. *Where there is a will, there is a way.*

Following is an incomplete but recent listing of forbidden drugs:

a) *Psychomotor stimulant drugs*
   e.g.
   amphetamine
   benzphetamine
   cocaine
   diethylpropion
   dimethylamphetamine
   ethylamphetamine
   fencamfamin
   methylamphetamine
   methylphenidate
   norspeudoephedrine
   phendimetrazine
   phenmetrazine
   prolintane
   and related compounds

b) *Sympathomimetic amines*
   e.g.
   ephedrine

methylephedrine
methoxyphenamine
and related compounds

c) *Miscellaneous central nervous system stimulants*
e.g.
amiphenazole
bemigride
leptazol
nikethamide
strychnine
and related compounds

d) *Narcotic analgesics*
e.g.
heroin
morphine
methadone
dextromoramide
dipipanone
pethidine
and related compounds

e) *Anabolic steroids*
e.g.
methandienone
stanozolol
oxymetholone
nandrolone decanoate
nandrolone phenylpropionate
and related compounds

A WORD ON TETANUS BOOSTERS

Accidents and sports injuries can all produce wounds that cause tetanus. In the past the medical practice dictated tetanus toxoid routinely in such wounds. This routine practice, however, may be unnecessary and in some instances actually harmful.

In the United States tetanus toxoid is the simplest, surest, and cheapest immunizing agent available and has achieved active immunization in most children and young adults. Many middle-aged and older men and women, however, have not been immunized, and this should always be taken into consideration.

Current practice in the United States is to begin active immunization early, usually before six months of age, and these infants will receive two or three intermuscular injections to protect them against various diseases, such as diphtheria, whooping cough and tetanus; they are usually given about 4 to 6 weeks apart, and then a booster is given when the child is usually a year old and another just before he enters school. While almost everyone agrees that booster injections are sometimes necessary, this question of giving them is still being argued and many studies have been done. As a result of these studies two changes from past practice are now accepted:

1. After accident immunization, routine boosters are no longer given at set intervals, and booster injections for routine wounds are considered unnecessary unless more than five years have elapsed since the last booster.

2. Of course, if the wound is particularly tetanus prone or treatment has been delayed and the wound looks bad and is soft and drains, a booster is needed if the patient has not received one in the preceding year.

Patients not previously immunized with tetanus toxoid should receive passive immunization at the time of injury. In the past physicians used equine or bovine antitoxin in doses of 1 to 500 to 1 to 3,000 units. Since allergic reactions occurred frequently, the antitoxin could not be given until skin tests or eye tests ruled out hypersensitivity. The passive protection was short-lived, usually lasting only 10 to 14 days, but the period of protection was even shorter if the patient had a previous history of horse-serum injection or showed any evidence of allergy.

But today these problems can be prevented by using tetanus immuno-globulin serum, which provides higher circulating antitoxin levels with lower doses and has much longer life, approximately 30 days. The routine prophylactic dose is 250 units. If the wound is particularly tetanus prone or if the debridement was delayed or inadequate, the dosage should be increased to 500 units.

Inasmuch as lifters handle iron and heavy weights and a bar might be rusty, they must be extra careful. If one injures his hand on a rusty bar, or injures his foot on a nail and hasn't had the immunization, he should certainly contact a physician immediately for a tetanus shot. It is also wise, when traveling abroad, to get immunized against typhoid, smallpox, cholera, and the like.

FIRST AID

ICE AND COLD TREATMENT

The application of ice to bruised or aching areas is an old but often misunderstood treatment. When one is bruised or bumped, it may not sound too good to apply cold to that area, but it certainly will help.

In acute trauma (pulling a ligament or tendon, tearing a muscle, spraining or separating a joint), or anywhere there is bruising of the surface or bleeding, blood will accumulate into the area as long as the blood's pressure has enough strength to push it into those tissues and will continue unless a counterpressure is applied.

Bleeding can be stopped in a number of ways, but the quickest and easiest is to apply an ice bag. In sports we spray a chemical agent known as ethyl chloride on the surface, and what appears to be frost accumulates on the area sprayed. This chilling effect tightens the blood vessels and stops any hemorrhaging; then we can apply an ice pack and pressure to the area to further stop the bleeding. Unless we can stop the bleeding in the area, the blood will accumulate and separate into clots and prevent the healing effort.

An ice bag should be applied for usually 12 to 24 hours. If there is a head injury, a turban can be tied around the head to hold the bag in position. If the bruising or the tear is deep—for example, in a hamstring in the back part of the thigh—be certain to apply extensive pressure and ice to the area. This was the case at the Montreal exhibition. Treated immediately, the young athlete was able to continue in the competition in one week and was very active and did well as a competitor. Had we not exerted pressure, blood would have accumulated in the area, and the clots would have stopped the healing, the serum may have accumulated, and a calcification may have developed in that area; the athlete may have been laid up for some period of time.

Sometimes a lifter tears the muscle below the knee, and the area is painful around the head of the fibula or along the big, heavy muscle at the back of the leg known as the gastrocnemius. He might even tear the fibers where the Achilles tendon is attached to this muscle. This will bleed down, and the individual will see black and blue around the right or left side of the Achilles tendon and into the ankle and may extend up along the side of the foot all the way up to the little toe, due to the hemorrhage bleeding and running down. This usually could have been prevented by using ice and a pressure bandage. Since this bleeding goes into the tissues, it takes considerable time for it to be absorbed and disables the athlete a longer period of time than usual. (*Note:* Be certain that the bandage is not too tight, causing paresthesia or numbness, especially around joints.)

When one has been lifting and preparing for a contest too extensively, lifting too many weights, he might develop a shoulder condition. The shoulder becomes rather irritated and painful due to excessive use, and the joint has become slightly irritated; there will be some secretion of fluids in the area. In this case an ice bag and pressure bandage are very beneficial to the area for a period of about 12 hours. In the afternoon it is wise to put the ice bag on with a pressure bandage over it. This goes under the shirt, and the lifter should not put his arm in his sleeve. He should wear this at least until he goes to bed, and at night he should apply a fresh, filled ice bag. Should he awaken during the night, he should fill the bag with fresh ice.

There are many products on the market that serve as substitutes for ice and cold applications, but still the most common course in our athletic procedure is actually using ice. Cold packs are made to be frozen and will stay that way for a long period of time. These are difficult to take out to the field with you, however, but if a refrigerator is in the gymnasium, the packs can be used and wrapped onto an affected area very easily.

As stated before, the use of ice (cold) is not new. When his feet were hot, bothered, and irritated, the first caveman probably cooled them in refreshing mountain streams. According to history, runners brought snow from the mountains to apply to the wounds of Alexander the Great after the battle of Gaugamela, and Caesar's legions considered cold water a prime treatment for wounds received in combat. If you had a nosebleed, your mother would apply an ice pack. Today we rely a lot on ice or cold, instead of drugs, to relieve pain, and in many cases cold reduces inflammation. Athletic trainers use an ice pack as a first-aid measure more often than anything else. Here's a great way to make your own ice pack: fill about a dozen styrofoam cups with water and place them in the deep freeze. Take them to meets, packing them in some dry ice if possible. When someone is injured, take one of the styrofoam cups of ice and cut the top half of the cup off, leaving the ice exposed. Then the ice can be applied without freezing one's hands; the styrofoam acts as insulation.

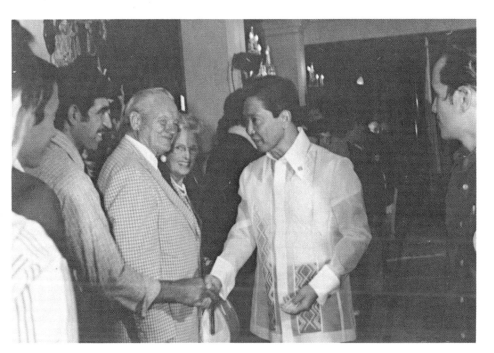

President Marcos (*center*)
of the Philippines, 1974

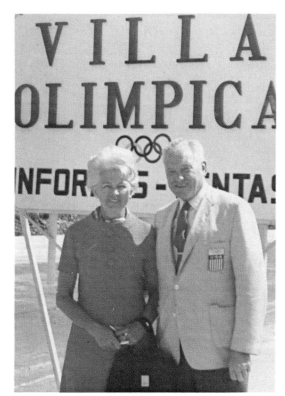

Dr. Wright and his
wife at the Mexican
Olympics, 1968

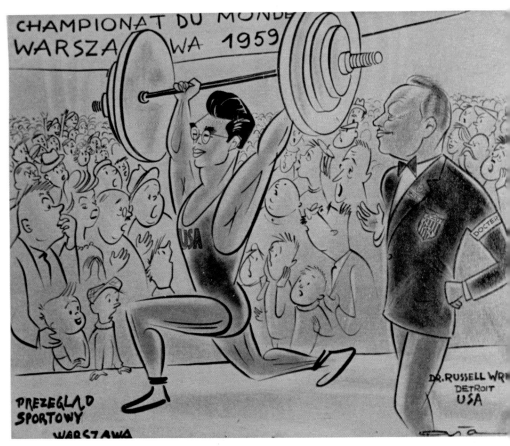

Poster from 1959 World Weight-Lifting Championships
in Warsaw, Poland

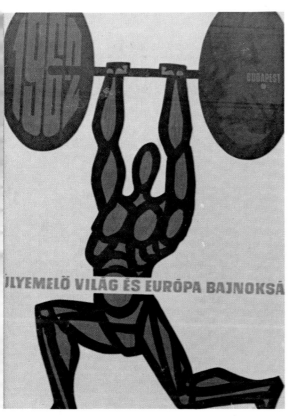

Poster from 1962 World
Weight-Lifting
Championships in Budapest,
Hungary

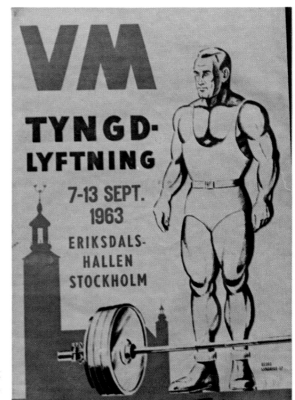

Poster from 1963 World
Weight-Lifting
Championships in Stockholm.
Sweden

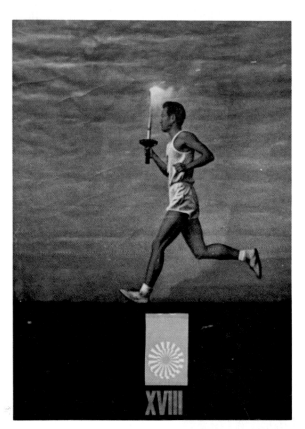

Poster from 1964 Olympics in Tokyo, Japan

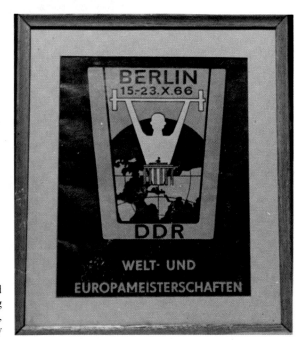

Poster from 1966 World Weight-Lifting Championships in Berlin, Germany

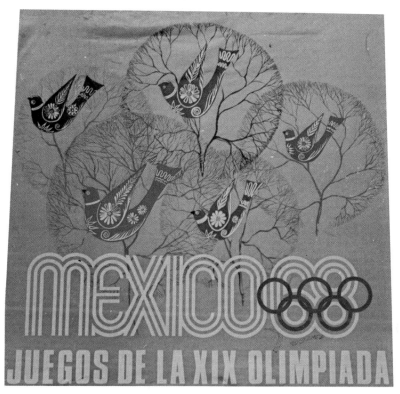

Poster from 1967 World Weight-Lifting Championships in Mexico

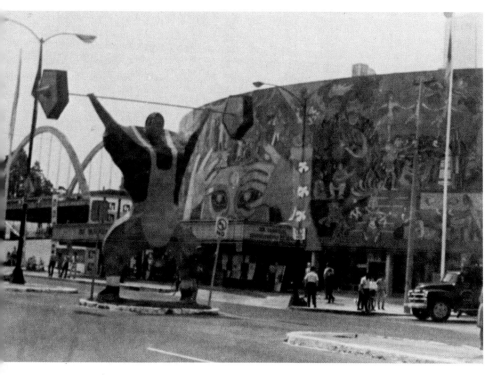

Papier-mache weight lifter guards entrance to stadium during
1968 Mexican Olympics

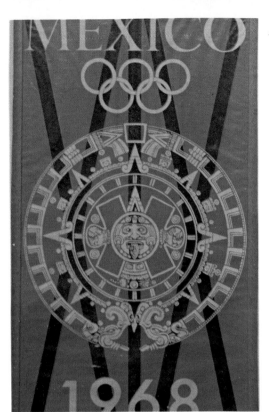

Poster from 1968 Olympics
in Mexico City, Mexico

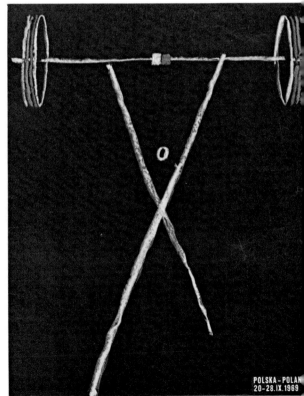

Poster from 1969 World
Weight-Lifting
Championships in Poland

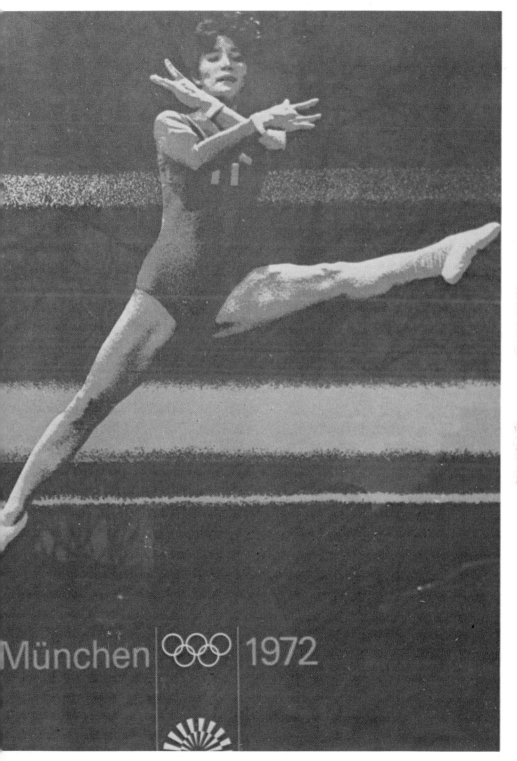

München 🟠 1972

Poster from 1972 Olympics in Munich, Germany

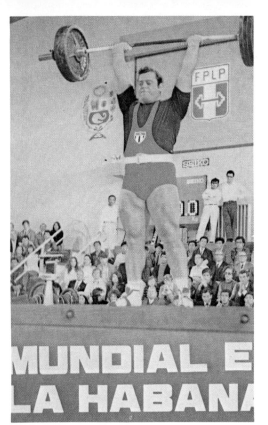

Poster from 1973 World Weight-Lifting Championships in Havana, Cuba

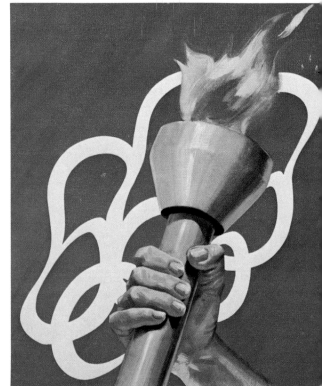

The 1976 Olympics, Montreal, Canada

W.F. MEDICAL COMMITTEE
EMBERS
(Not pictured) Dr. M. Ono, Dr. V. nadze

Russell Wright, President
(photo courtesy of Storer-Spellan)

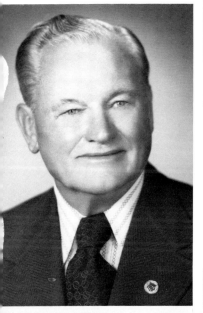

Dr. G. Georgiev

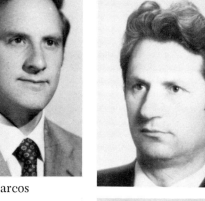

Dr. J. Marcos

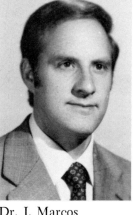

Dr. M. Sadeghi

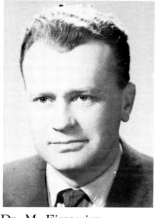

Dr. M. Firsowicz

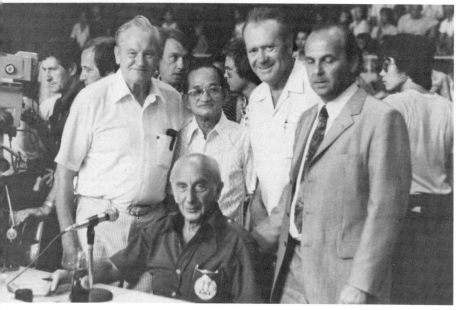

From left to right: Dr. Wright, unidentified, Dr. Firsowicz, G. Schodl (president of I.W.F.), and *(seated)* Oscar State (executive secretary of I.W.F.)

From left to right: Dr. Wright, Fauquez (Belgian heavyweigh
and André Dupont (Belgian national coach)

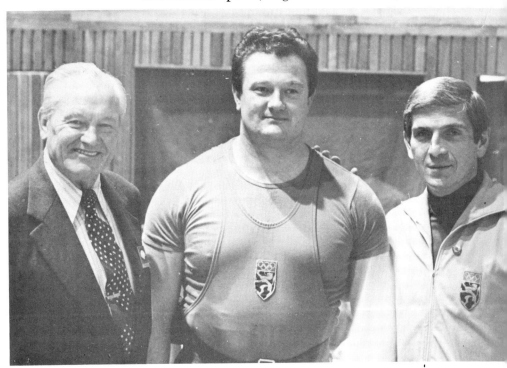

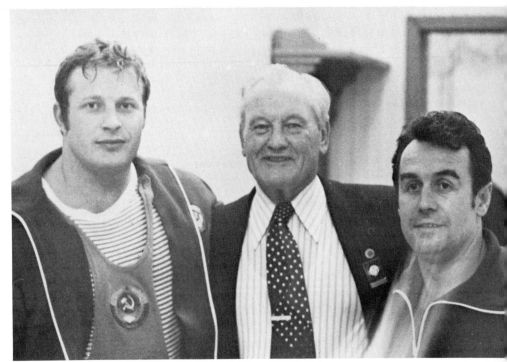

From left to right: Vasili Mozheikov (U.S.S.R. heavyweight),
Wright, and Igor Kudyukov (Russian national coach)

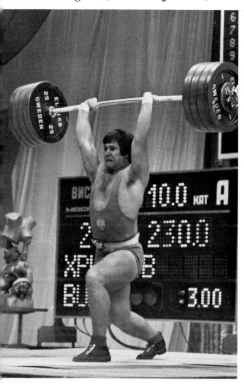

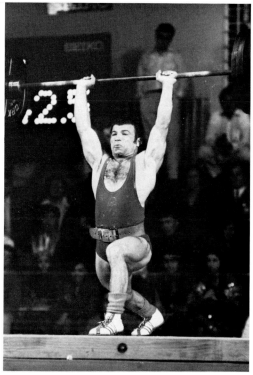

Mohamud Vassiri, Lima, Peru, 1971 *(Bob Berry Photo)*

Vasili Alexeev, U.S.S.R., world record holder *(Bob Berry Photo)*

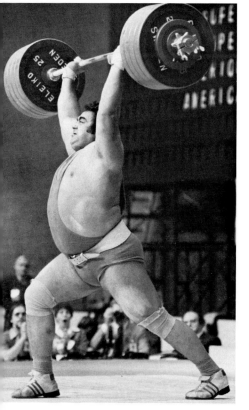

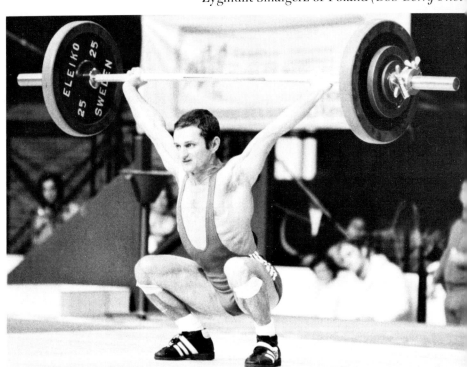

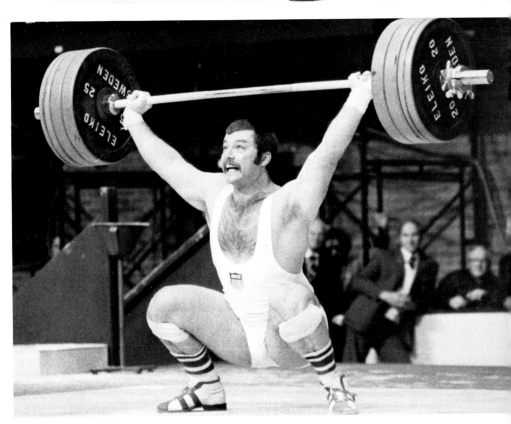

Mark Cameron, U.S.A. *(Bob Berry Pho*

. Wright and Bob Bednarski

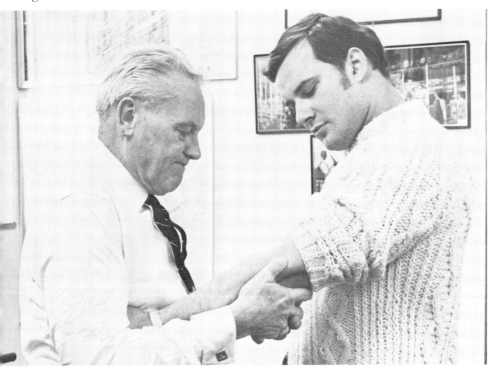

Norbert
Schemansky

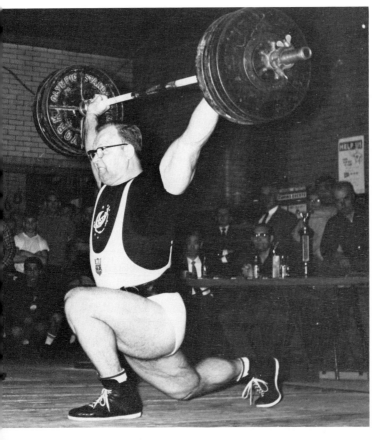

Tommy Kono

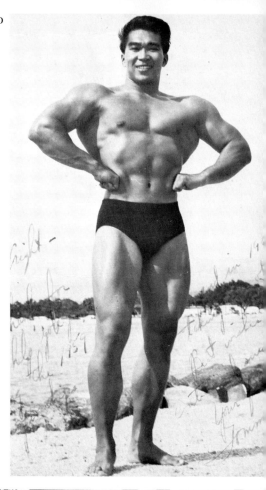

From left to right: Bo Johannson, Clarence Johnson, Dr. Richard Wright, Don Graham, and Dr. Wright

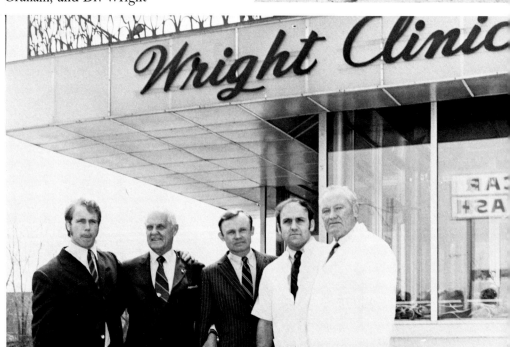

om left to right: Dr. Wright, Olympic coach Bob Hoffman, rld champion Norbert Schemansky, and Clarence Johnson, norary I.W.F. president (photo taken at 1964 Olympics in *an)

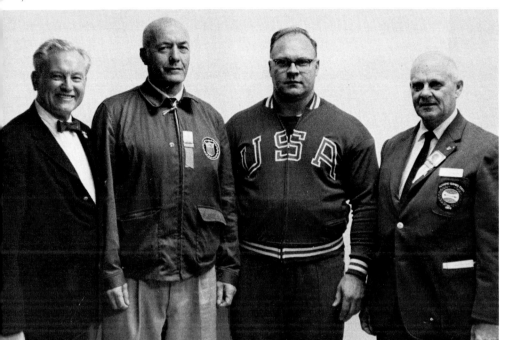

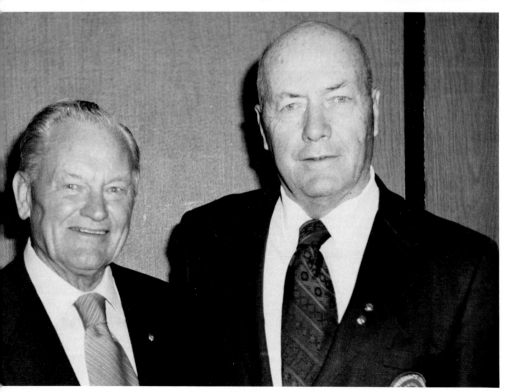

r. Wright *(left)* and Olympic coach Bob Hoffman

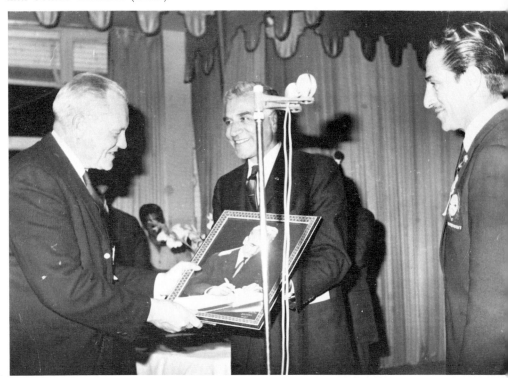

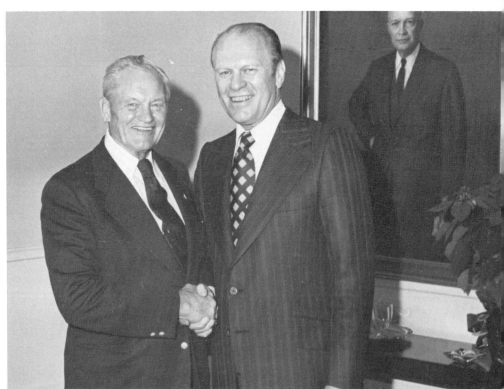

Dr. Wright and President Gerald Ford

BURNS

When someone has been burned, a basic knowledge of first aid can mean the difference between life and death.

First, determine what caused the burn. Maybe the victim will be able to tell you or someone who may have been present. Was it caused by a flame, say from a torch or match? Maybe it's a chemical burn, an electrical burn, or a thermal burn (scalding water, steam, hot tar, hot grease, or hot syrups).

Now that you have determined the cause, determine how badly the skin was burned. There are first-, second-, and third-degree burns.

A first-degree burn is characterized by irritation of the skin surface. It might be pink, it's painful to the touch, and this burn is often caused by prolonged exposure to sunlight. Usually there is no blistering, but this type of burn is painful, though mild.

A second-degree burn is very painful. It too can be caused by sunburn; the skin becomes very red; there may be some swelling (edema) and blistering. The surface of the skin is usually moist and painful. If the skin has not been broken, this type of burn heals rather readily in 10 to 14 days.

The third-degree burn is much more severe. Instead of the skin surface being moist, it is dry and has a white, burned or charred appearance. It may not be painful because the nerve endings have been destroyed. This patient eventually may need a skin graft. If this patient is burned badly about the eyes, they should be protected, and if burned about the mouth and throat, it might be necessary to use an airway so that the patient can breathe. Every coach or trainer on every field where sports activity is performed should have an airway available.

If possible, move the individual to the most comfortable place you can, providing it's close by, and place ice or cold water over the wound. The ice should be wrapped or applied in an ice bag, not directly to the skin. It is best to have sterile dressings; if you do not have these, use a clean piece of sheet or cloth. Place that over the skin and saturate with cold water or apply ice bag.

Remember to put ice in an ice bag. Don't apply it directly to the wound because it may cause more damage. There should be a layer of cloth between the ice and the skin.

With the possible exception of first-degree-burn cases, second- and third-degree victims should be removed to a hospital as soon as possible. The amount of skin surface burned many times determines the severity of the burn and the victim's chances of survival, so respond immediately to give the patient relief. See that he can breathe and give him something for his pain—an analgesic, aspirin, codeine, or whatever the trainer is using for pain and is available.

WORDS OF CAUTION

Don't apply heat directly to the testicular area or immediately following an injury, unless you are sure that internal bleeding has stopped.

Don't demand performance to the detriment of the athlete.

Be sure to maintain a healthy water and salt balance.

Don't massage an infected area or wound.

Don't leave an unconscious athlete unattended.

Don't allow an athlete to participate if he is feverish.

Section VII

SPEAKING FROM EXPERIENCE

TOMORROW IS THE CHANCE
AT THE BLUE RIBBON

What changes does the young man undergo? What does he think about? What must he do? Well, first he worries about his weight. If he is overweight, he knows that he will be eliminated from the contest—this is called not making weight. In order to make weight, some athletes try to lose 5 to 6 lbs. in one day, which is not the easiest thing to do without its having some effect. During competition or practice, it is undesirable for the athlete to lose more than 5 percent of his body weight; in other words, if he weighs 200 lbs., he shouldn't lose more than 10 lbs. because he may go into shock, or, if he's outside in the hot sun, he may develop sunstroke. This is the guideline we follow.

Tomorrow the boy has a chance to win a medal. If there is a tie, the boy weighing the least in his division will be given the blue ribbon. So it is important to watch the weight. If an athlete is a few pounds overweight, he's going to have to sit in a steam bath, exercise, cut down his fluids and food—whatever is necessary for him to meet the weight requirements. In the last few years, some of these young men have resorted to taking diuretics, which increase urination and the dehydration of body tissues. This is a bad policy. I have seen these same individuals go into competition, make the weight, get hold of the bar, maybe even make it up into position and make the lift, but, because of the terrific pressure on their hands, fail to hold that weight for a period of a few seconds because their hands went into a spasm, and someone had to actually pull their hands and remove them from the bar. Because the blood supply was cut down, athletes would develop a muscle spasm of this nature. The muscles of one's back may also be affected this way. One should be prepared, knowing which weight class he's going to make by starting a week in advance, not two days before a meet, to get down to where he can make weight. Most good weight lifters know what they can do and how fast they lose weight, but don't overshoot your gun and lose too much weight in the last 24 hours, and don't resort to diuretics; they might cost you that blue ribbon.

The second thing an athlete faces is tension and possible hyperventilation. He is waiting to be called for his first lift, he's somewhat excited, and he's sitting back on a bench. As he watches the others go before him, he knows his turn is coming up, he's becoming a little more anxious, a little more nervous. The next thing he knows, he finds himself sliding over to the edge of the bench, then being up on his toes, and holding the edge of the bench with his fingertips. His breathing becomes a little deeper, a little deeper, and soon he is taking in good, deep breaths and then blowing them out—shooooooooooooooooo, another deep breath—shooooooooooo. Next he becomes dizzy and can hardly stand, and it's his turn to lift. What has happened to him? He has exhaled too much carbon dioxide; quickly cup your hands over his mouth (a paper bag is better if available) and let him breathe into it so that he inhales his own carbon dioxide. Within a minute he will be able to do his lift.

The third thing I've seen happen to these boys occurs at the very last moment. They are warming up and practicing, and sometimes when we've moved to a different place for maybe the final night for the weight lifting to allow for a larger crowd of people, the weather might be inclement and the new gym area is cold. The temperature may have dropped down to 45° or 50°, and it is difficult to keep the athlete warm. He may get a bit of a muscle spasm, a charley horse or a lumbar spasm, if he doesn't cover up. This spasm may be so great that it pulls him down, and he's bent to one side and can't straighten up. He's due to go on in a minute's time. He's worked all his life to be at the Olympics, and now is his chance to win, to be first and best in the world, and now he's got a pain and he can't stand up straight, let alone lift. I have worked out a treatment, as this is not an uncommon condition (see figs. 55a, 55b, 55c). Standing back to back, slip your arms through the athlete's arms, and then bend over and pick him up on your back. Rotate from right to left (if it is his right side that is tight with spasm), hitting him with your left hip in the right sacroiliac as you pull him up, bending forward, and have him stretched, lying on your back. Usually that muscle will respond and let go. Then he can go in and pick up the weight. That happened to Martin in Great Britain, and within the next few minutes he had won the World Championship, and my treatment helped. Otherwise his lifetime goal would have been cancelled out immediately.

As all are getting ready and becoming nervous after hours of waiting, many things have been suggested for the boys to do. Some of them drink tea, some coffee, some Coca-Cola; others want to eat some kind of food. The energy burned up is extremely heavy, and I find that it seemed to help these individuals to put honey in hot tea as a supplement to give them energy, and it can be converted into energy very quickly, especially in the boy who has had trouble making weight and has been cutting his food and fluids to make weight.

OLYMPIC PARTICIPATION

I would like to participate on the Olympic team. I think I could win a gold medal. There are about 10,000 athletes from all over the world competing in the various Olympic sports, one of which is weight lifting.

You must be the best athlete in the world that day to win the gold medal. Yes, there is a winner and it can be you. One does not wish himself into the position of Olympic participant or gold-medal winner—he earns it. He starts out working, training, listening to his coach, his parents, his trainer, his doctor, reading the many fine writings, and accepting any advice that he can procure to help him. Many of us expect to be successful immediately and may be, due to our coordination, natural ability and observation. Then we slip and wonder why. Success requires training over and over and over again. Yes, it can be fun, too, but never lose sight of your goal, for that gold medal can be yours.

First you win the school meet in your weight class, getting used to those blue ribbons; then the inner school and the county or district or the state meet; then the sectionals for your area of the country; then you will be invited to an invitational: you will go to the nationals; finally you will be selected by your country to participate in the Olympics.

You will have a period of special training; special clothes are designed for the Olympic teams and special shoes, along with particular types of bags in which to carry your clothing. This is all selected for the national team participating in the greatest of all athletic events. You will meet boys and girls from all over the world. You will understand their smiles, their laughs, and their tears, but how wonderful if you could speak several languages. Think what an ambassador of goodwill you would be for your nation, for you have been chosen as one of the world's finest young athletes—all of a sudden, there you are; you are the selectee. It makes no difference if you are from the most humble home in one of the poorest sections of the nation, or whether you are from one of the wealthiest families, or a metropolitan area, or the finest district in your country— you have arrived at the Olympics. You represent your nation's fairness, thoughtfulness, kindness, and strength; and your very presence can aid world peace.

You will arrive with your fellow teammates at our place in the Olympic Village. You are breathless—there's so much to see, do, and

117

hear about. As you walk about and train, you can think of nothing but victory, and then you dream of it at night. The opening day of the Olympics you line up with your particular team and the other teams of the nations. All the teams of the world march into this great amphitheater where 80,000 people are looking down and cheering as you are entering this great stadium. Your top athlete will probably be carrying the Olympic flag and your country's flag, and all the great athletes of your nation will be lined up behind him.

The first banner and emblem or plaque will be that of Greece, as that was the home of the first Olympics, and then the countries will line up in alphabetical order, the last one being the host nation. As you line up and come into the stadium you start in the center of the field and work both ways till all this great mass of the world's greatest athletes are lined up, facing the reviewing stand. Then the Olympic flag will be flown, and a torchbearer will come through the gate and into the stadium, around the track, up into the top of the stands, and touch the torch to the great light—the eternal flame of the Olympics is lit. Hundreds of pigeons are released from cages all around the stadium, and they fly to all the various parts of the nation announcing the Olympiad has begun.

You have seen and heard so much in a short time that your eyeballs are sore and your mental recording equipment taxed to the utmost, but tomorrow is when you come in and make a run for the goal. Tomorrow your competition begins, and all your dreams and efforts are expanded to make your run for the gold.

THE AMATEUR ATHLETE
AND THE OLYMPICS

Much has been said about the classification of athletes as amateurs or professionals. As we set up our athletic programs from one country to another, we find the system of classification differs with each government. Here in America paid athletes are considered professionals: their sport is their employment. Amateurs are not paid and train on their own time. In other countries, where everyone works for the government, the individual seemingly has more time to train, and since he is working for the government he is supported by it. So an athlete considered an amateur in America may not be considered an amateur somewhere else, and the question of fair competition arises.

We are certain that in those countries where sports are government sponsored the athlete has a better life economically, better athletic equipment and training facilities than he does in most of the democratic countries, where the individual works and finds it difficult for him to be relieved from his work to train and take care of his family and to prepare for and attend national meets and the Olympic Games.

It's no wonder the Olympics are no longer a sign of world peace, but rather a commercialized bout for gold. John B. Kelly, Jr., A.A.U. president, made such note in the following excerpt from an article printed in the *A.A.U. News* (vol. 43, no. 10, October 1972):

The founder of the modern Olympiad, Baron de Coubertin, personified the spirit of the Olympic Games with the statement, "It is not the winning, but the taking part that counts." However, in this modern era, the Games would be better characterized by the cynical expression, "It is not whether you win or lose—it's whether you win!"

It is, then, not so much that the Olympic Games now need restructuring; they have always needed restructuring. It is not that they are now too large; it's that they always had the aura of the colossus surrounding them. It is not that they now provoke political behavior; it's just that we have never admitted the rampant political activity that has always gone on in the Games.

What will be required (in fact, what is being demanded by Congress right now) will be new innovations to minimize some of the

problems of the Games. Perhaps, as has been suggested in the Legis-
lative branch, a restructuring of the Olympic Committee will be
necessary. It is, as I have suggested in the past, perhaps a necessity to
bring more and more athletes into the decision-making process with
regard not only to our sports, but also to Olympic participation. And,
in line with this, we must determine that financial limitations do not
preclude these athlete representatives from attending meetings where
policy is decided.

Perhaps, too, as has been suggested, we should push for a new
format of the Games. Among the many suggestions is that we eliminate
national anthems, that athletes march and dress according to their
sport rather than according to their country, and that we make the
Games smaller by switching some of the sports that are now in the
Summer Games to the Winter Games. Additionally, it has been suggested that separate World Championships be held in each individual
sport. This would effectively reduce the size of the Olympic Games.
Then, during the quadrennium these individual competitions would
be classified as the Olympics of that sport.

Overriding the entire change in the structure, though, should be
this thought: we need to get back to the true Olympic spirit. We
have spent, it seems to me, too much time wondering whether a man
is an "amateur" or not, and not enough time concerning ourselves with
the spirit behind his competition in the Olympic Games. What should
be pervasive in our thinking in these matters is relevancy of the
Games to a modern era. We cannot adapt this era to the Games, so
we must adapt the Games to the era.

CONTACT SPORTS
AT JUNIOR-HIGH LEVEL

When one considers the preadolescent or adolescent boy, one must consider his psychic makeup—one minute forgetful, listless, inconsiderate and carefree; the next a world beater. He will listen to every suggestion made to him and carry it out to the best of his ability. He must have instilled in him the desire to win, which carries with it the desire to get into and stay in shape. He must have this urging to get in shape or he will never do it. It naturally follows that if the boy is not in shape his team will not very likely win, and, more important, he is much more prone to injury. Sam Bishop, well-known Detroit Northwestern High coach, and Jesse Owens attest to the importance of conditioning.

Why are boys injured when not in condition? Because of FATIGUE. This is a physiologic reaction in the muscles, which accumulate lactic acid during exercise, producing fatigue. Conditioning creates better blood supply, reduces fatigue, and, therefore, lessens injury.

Much has been suggested relative to the physical examination. A questionnaire we have found helpful for use by coaches and filled out by candidates for his team gives early information to the coach and starts the boys thinking about conditioning:

1. Weight, height and age
2. Measurement—mid calf, mid thigh and one inch above knee
3. Chest measurement on inspiration and expiration
4. Time to run: 100 yards, ¼ mile, ½ mile, mile
5. Number of push-ups
6. Number of times he can chin himself
7. Yards he can throw and kick a football
8. Feet he can broad jump
9. Feet he can high jump
10. Nickname or name he prefers to be called

Clues to certain leg problems can be detected by this review. I have always admired the great athlete Jack Adams of the Detroit Red Wings Hockey Club, who said, "Great legs and great teams go hand in hand."

It is important in these youngsters to consider the selection of adequate equipment. The proper fitting of his equipment—helmet, shoes, jockstrap, shoulder pads, etc.—will save many disabling injuries that can cause anxiety and regrets the rest of the boy's life. We must keep in mind that he is not just a junior high lad; he is the scholastic varsity material of tomorrow and, in turn, college material—Olympic athlete and future leader of our community and nation. The choosing of a dependable boy interested to help in this area and under the coach's supervision is a great aid to the coach.

TEAM BALANCE

One must study the biological age of the participants, always thinking of protection from injury as well as those problems common to the boys' level of growth. Always observe for any abnormal symptoms and seek medical opinion. It is not uncommon to see cases of unrecognized serious injury permitted to go unchecked due to lack of close observation and consultation. Good judgment saves much anxiety, suffering, and disability. Where indicated, follow-up care must be required, including blood and urine tests, x-ray evaluation, and periodic reexamination of the injured player. If the coach or physician is not satisfied with the boy's appearance, or if the trouble cannot be located, consultation should be sought.

IMPORTANCE OF OFFICIATING

One of the most important problems in the reduction of injury is to have good officiating. These boys must know that they cannot clip, trip, or hold without paying the penalty. They must learn to play the game fairly and that anything less will not be tolerated. The coach must insist on fair play. Every boy must know it, appreciate it, and respect it.

CONSERVATIVE USE OF THE HANDICAPPED

In any school system there are boys who long to be part of the finest segment of an American boy's life—athletics—but are not physically able to compete on the same level with the average boys. What can be done for them? Much! What is the difference if a group of five boys race in times of 20 seconds or 11 seconds. It is a good race. You are giving the handicapped the honor, the pride of playing and winning. They must be included.

I know that many times you may say to yourself, "I am but one, what can I do?" To quote Circuit Court Judge Edward Piggins, "My answer is that history shows repeatedly that one man can start a wave of action, that leadership of strong moral men will call forth the power of the people, the true power of the nation." *Remember the greatest use of life is spending it for something that will outlast you.*

Dr. Wright and his son, Richard

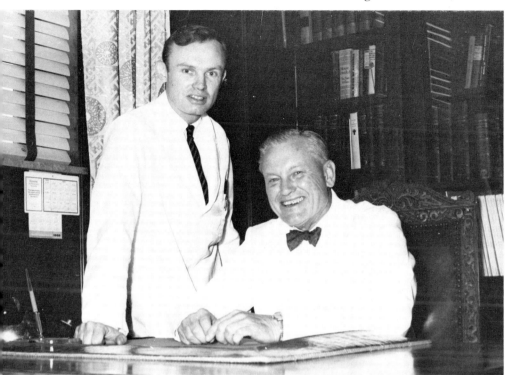

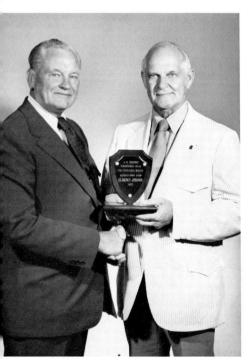

arence Johnson *(right)* presents Dr.
'right with the A. W. Thompson Award
r his contributions to sports *(Photo cour-
sy of Storer-Spellman)*

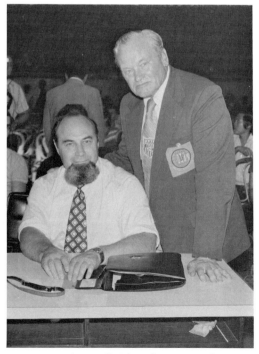

Dr. A. Yorobyev *(left)* and Dr. Wright

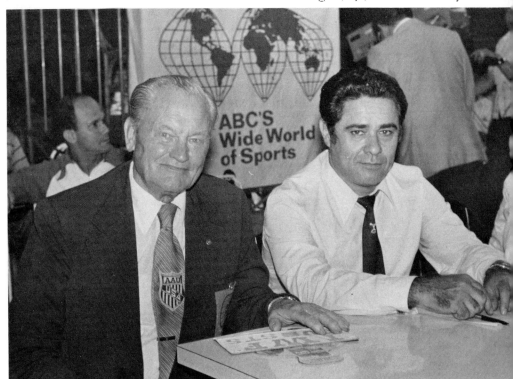

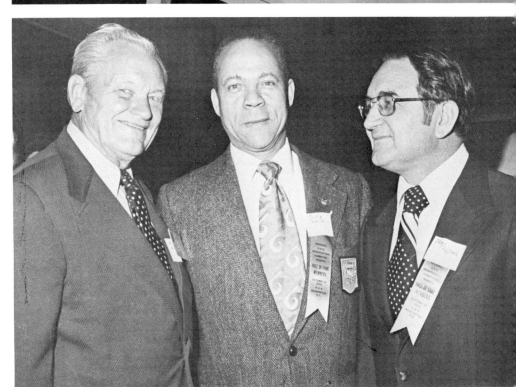

From left to right: Dr. Wright, and Weight-Lifting Hall-
Famers Rudy Sablo and John Terpak

r. and Mrs. Wright are welcomed to the Philippines by E. S.
orothea, vice-president of the I.W.F.

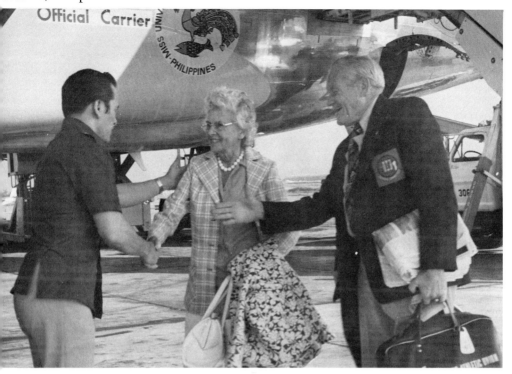

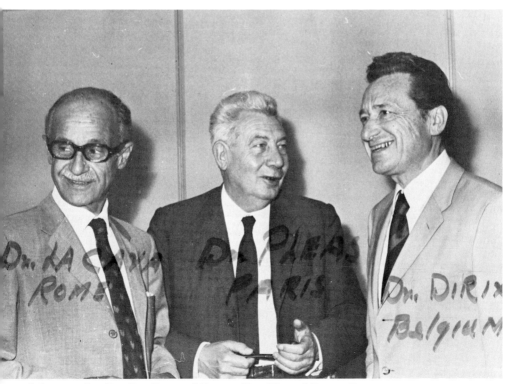

om left to right: Dr. La Cava of Rome, Dr. Plas of Paris, Dr.
irix of Belgium (photo taken in 1973 in Madrid)

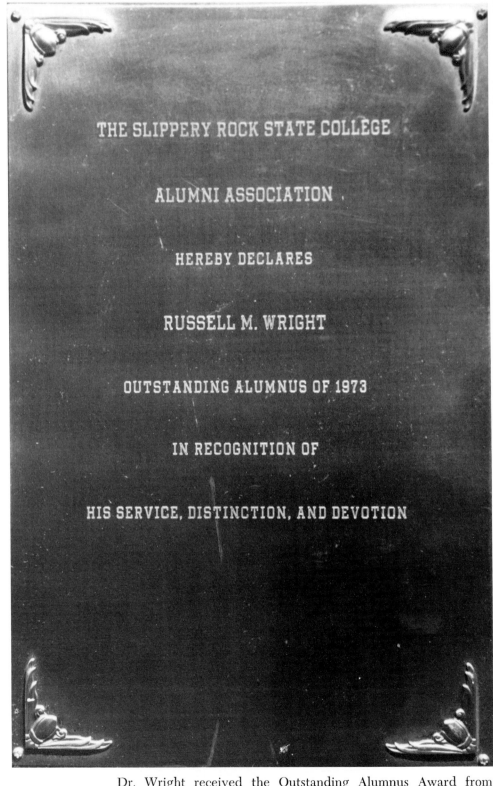

THE SLIPPERY ROCK STATE COLLEGE

ALUMNI ASSOCIATION

HEREBY DECLARES

RUSSELL M. WRIGHT

OUTSTANDING ALUMNUS OF 1973

IN RECOGNITION OF

HIS SERVICE, DISTINCTION, AND DEVOTION

Dr. Wright received the Outstanding Alumnus Award from Slippery Rock State College for fifty years' contribution to sports

A: R. M. WRIGHT

MIEMBRO DEL COMITE MEDICO
DE LA I. W. F.

COMO RECUERDO DEL cuba/73

XXVII Campeonato Mundial y I Panamericano
de Levantamiento de Pesas

Federación Nacional Amateur de
Levantamiento de Pesas de Cuba

Dr. Wright was given an award by the Cuban government for
his contribution to sports in that country

World-Championship medals
awarded to Dr. Wright

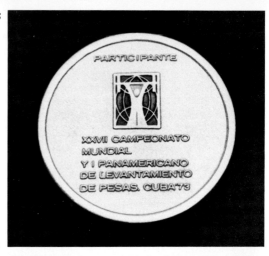

CUBA

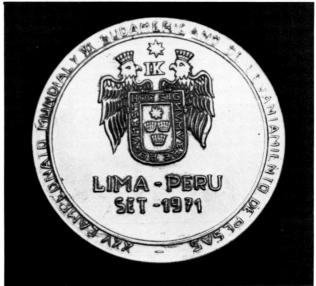

PERU

TEHRAN

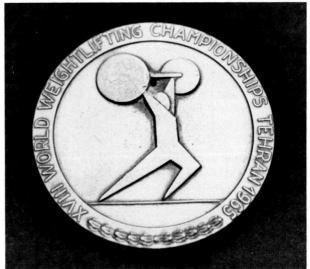

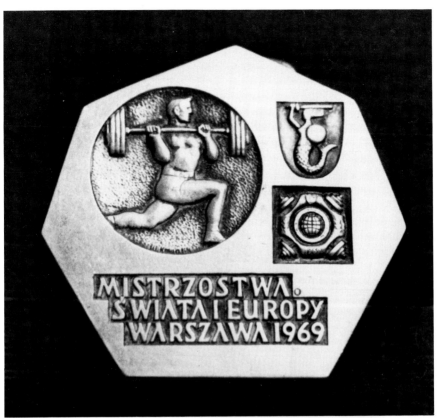

POLAND

U.S.S.R.

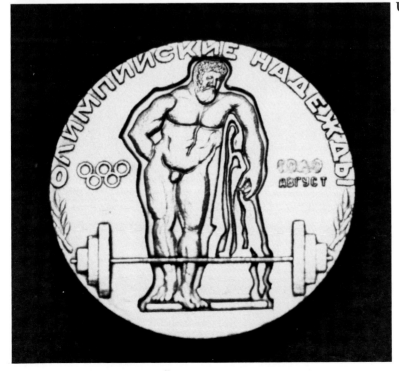

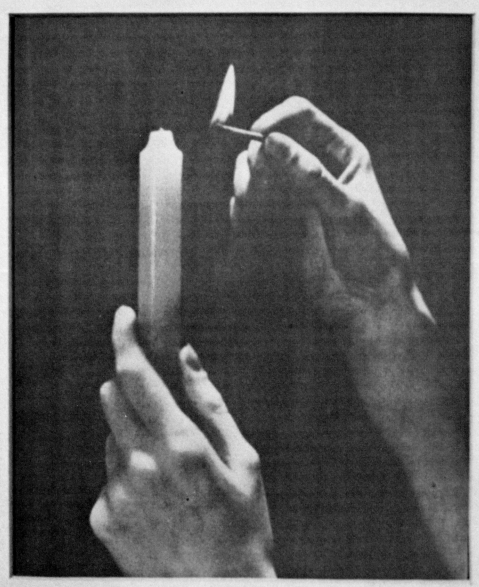

'It is better to light a candle
than to curse the darkness'

This picture was given to Dr. Wright by his mother. It has been
a source of inspiration to him over the years.

AN INTERVIEW WITH MORRIS WEISSBROT

QUESTIONS AND ANSWERS

What is the difference between weight training and weight lifting?

Weight training and lifting use progressive resistance exercises to develop the body. Now, weight lifting is a scientific sport which has to be engaged in under very stringent rules—the rules of competition. You can be a weight-training athlete for many years without ever having gone into weight lifting. Weight lifting only involves those recognized movements which we have written rules for. It doesn't have to be the two Olympic lifts. Years ago we had competition on a lot of one-hand lifts and so-called odd lifts which, of course, we call power lifts. Anybody can do weight training, but not everyone wants to do weight lifting. Weight lifting is trying to lift more and more, either competing with yourself or against the standard, whereas with weight training, all you do is use exercises to develop parts of the body.

Most colleges and universities have weight-training programs as a basis for all their sports. When we held our intercollegiate championships, we had as many as thirty-three different colleges competing. We are trying to get it recognized as a letter sport in a lot of colleges so that we can get scholarships. Some colleges will give a letter for weight lifting. For example, Cornell University gives a letter, Southern Methodist University gives a letter, and Texas Christian gives a letter. A youngster, say in grade school, is a fantastic prospect—he can't look forward to an athletic scholarship the way he could if he were a track star or a basketball star.

When would you start a boy into weight lifting or weight training?

I would start a boy into weight training at about the age of puberty, 13 or 14—around those years. I wouldn't start him any sooner. I'd let him do the normal things, like running, rough-and-tumble sports, perhaps rope-skipping. Now weight lifting has begun at 12 and 13 with our Junior Olympic Program, but I'm not really in favor of it.

Have you seen any of them develop epiphysitis from injury to any of the joints?

Not from weight lifting, no, but the way I look at it, most of these fellows, even the ones who are into Junior Olympics, have had enough basic body-building movements and enough basic weight-training movements so that the joints have tightened sufficiently, and they have built up enough tissue around the joint area. Now, we still have some occasions where a fellow's elbow will dislocate, mostly in the young boys trying to hold a snatch overhead, for example, because the joints are just not strong enough. That's why I'm against limited tests for these really young fellows.

Well, when you start a boy—we'll say you are going to start him at 13 or 14—what lifts are we going to do? A bench press?

First of all, I think the boy should develop the lower back, the hips, the thighs, and I would start him off with things like deep knee bends, some repetition bend lifts to develop the lower back, shoulders, overhead presses. The bench press? I don't think that is important in the beginning. It's a good movement, but I wouldn't emphasize it too much because— what happens there—as the boy gets into it, he finds that he can very rapidly add weight to the bench press, add poundage to the bar, so he starts to overdo it, and the next thing you know he has overdeveloped pectoral muscles, and his chest cavity hasn't really expanded, but the pectorals have become very, very strong. The tendency is, therefore, to get that scoop-chested look. The pectorals are big and strong, but are actually bowing the shoulders forward. I have seen this in some fellows.

These big linemen that we get in here develop terrific pectorals, and they haven't come up in the back, and they get a caveman look with a curvature that is not really natural.

This happens quite frequently to a young fellow. The tendency is to develop those muscles that he can see, and a lot of these fellows like to train in front of a mirror. They look at the muscles, and they can see their pectorals, but they can't see the large muscles of the back, for instance, the rhomboid, scapula, the whole area around the lower back, especially the most important set of muscles in the human body, to my way of thinking.

What other exercises when he is doing this? What about jumping rope? And running in place?

Running in place and jumping rope should continue on, even if a fellow has had 12 or 13 years under his belt. He should continue this, as you know, for the cardiovascular reserve. You know this.

I also believe in a lot of stretching; the flexibility work is so important. The muscles have to go from fullest extent of contraction to fullest extent of flexion. It's got to go over the whole range of movement, otherwise you have an incomplete development there, which so often happens in the body builder. The reason I emphasize stretching, I tell people—you talk about being physically fit, agile, and strong, but did you ever see a cat lift weights or do pushups? Yet a cat is tremendously agile. What does a cat do? The first thing it does on rising is stretch; it stretches in many directions. Right? The human body is also designed to stretch, so I say we must do a lot of stretching. When I work with my lifters, that is one of the things I insist on—a lot of stretching. As you stretch more and more, you will find that you will become less liable to injury.

When you say stretching, do you mean reaching as high as you can into the air?

Reaching up is only one form of stretching. When I say *stretching,* I mean, for example, stretching the hamstrings—sitting on the floor, spreading the feet wide apart, bending forward to touch the floor, having your hands touch your toes, with the legs perfectly straight. There are all kinds of stretching. When I say *stretching,* I mean stretching the hamstrings, the calves, the ankles, the shoulders, everything.

How do you stretch the ankles?

There are several ways. Number one, walk up close to a wall, and put your toe up against the wall at a 45° angle, and press down very hard. Another way is to keep your palms flat against the wall, and then back away from it, keeping the legs straight, so there is a stretch right there.

To strengthen the wrist, take a bar, add a rope on it with a weight— say, a couple of pounds—and then roll it up and roll it back down.

When a boy comes in, how long would you train him if he's 12 or 13 years old? How long can you keep his attention in training? Would you give him 15 minutes of jumping rope and running in place?

An absolute beginner—I'd give him about 5 to 10 minutes of the preliminaries; then I'd put him through about 5 to 10 minutes of exercise movements with an empty bar. Just let him learn what it's all about.

A broom handle?

A broom handle, right. A broom handle is one of the best training aids we have.

Would you have him do deep squats with this and go down and lightly bounce his buttocks against his heels, if he can?

Yes, that would be good. Not everybody can do this. Some fellows will go down with a rush, and even with no weight there is a crunching effect on the knee, so I prefer to go down at a slow and controlled pace. You always have to stretch flat back, head erect, shoulders up. Don't ever let the boy bow his back.

Make him stay straight?

Right, until it becomes a habit. He can handle more weight with the back rounded. That's why a lot of lifters do it, but it's dangerous.

What about preparation of a fellow's hands? Is there any way? I notice they go in there and powder their hands. The kids starting on the bar, I think it was Moscow, were all tearing their hands, and we changed the bar. Is there anything we should look for in a boy's hands? Some of them tear easier. Is there any way to harden them?

A lot of fellows allow calluses to build up. The best thing to do is to keep the palms completely uncalloused, use a little emery cloth, sandpaper or pumice stone, and work on it everyday. The skin becomes toughened, but then you don't have that tremendous callus built up. Calluses tear because of the build up under the skin, and when they grab the bar the pressure actually rips that mass away from the rest of the hands. But if you eliminate the mass, you eliminate the danger, so I believe in emery cloth, sandpaper. I also believe in hand lotion. A little soft skin cream, lanolin at night. Gymnasts do this, and they certainly take a far greater beating on their hands.

After these boys have worked out, I notice some, when taking a shower, will stay in there forever; others just soap in a hot shower and then a cool shower and out. What's your thinking on that?

Well, sometimes a fellow actually will need a long, hot shower. If he's had a hard workout, he really needs that little extra relaxation. The hot water is beneficial. It does have a good effect on tired muscles. Let's face it, it feels good to stand under the shower and rub yourself down. There is nothing wrong with a quick shower, but some fellows take it too quickly. They take a cold shower, which is a chill to the body, and it's definitely a shock to the body by the closing of blood vessels.

Jesse Owens, the winner of all the medals in Germany in 1936, felt that a lot of energy might be lost by staying too long in the hot shower.

I agree with him, because it has a definite enervation effect. Let's face it, if you relax in a nice, warm tub, you are not going to feel very peppy when you get out. The same thing with a long, hot shower. It is enervating because the body is actually expending energy just to maintain its normal temperature under those conditions.

If these boys are really sore after a workout and so on, as far as drugs, do you give them aspirin or anything, or do they just work it out?

A little massage and they work it out.

What about anabolic steroids?

I am dead set against them. They are the worst curse of mankind. You know, these fellows think the only way they are going to get to the top is with anabolic steroids. Most of it is psychological. You can get the same effect with sugar pills or placebos. There may be some beneficial effects. We don't know what. But I don't think those effects are worth the risk, because the side effects become too horrendous. You get an athlete who destroys himself with anabolic steroids. He may become a great champion with the use of the drugs, and then he wears a peanut shell and a rubber band for a jockstrap the rest of his life because his testicles are atrophied. I don't consider it worth it. You're an athlete only a few years, but you've got to be a man a long time.

I heard the president of the A.A.U. say that sometimes there's a boy who's 115, 120, or 125 lbs., and when he goes and asks for a football suit, the coach tells him to get lost, and he becomes incorrigible. He raises hell in school, and it's found that he is failing in school and may be one of the people who ends up in jail. But if they had had a course in boxing, wrestling, or weight lifting, the guy might have been a good, top athlete and been a fine individual. Do you concur on that?

I certainly do. Every person wants to excel at something. It's natural, normal. A young kid or even an older fellow in his twenties—if he's small and slight of stature and slight of build—his bone structure is such that he'll never weigh more than 120 lbs. in his life, and he certainly is never going to play football. He can't realize his dreams as a great athlete, but in certain sports that small size is an asset, sports like weight lifting, boxing, and wrestling. Now, I don't like boxing and wrestling too much because I don't like contact sports. There's one thing about weight lifting —*the weights don't ever hit you back*. I find that it becomes a self-testing thing. You can actually gauge your progress from day to day, week to week, month to month, and this to me is a source of tremendous self-satisfaction. Of course, when you develop a competition spirit in some of these fellows, then they find that they are competing against their peers, guys their own size, their own weight, and their own age, and this is something they would never enjoy any other way. So I agree with Joe Scalso [A.A.U. president] definitely and wholeheartedly.

There has been so much said about diets, vitamins, and food supplements, and so on; from your experience in your lifetime in this work what do you think about these?

Well, doctors have always told us that you get nutritional needs from your daily diet. You, as a doctor, know what your average diet is— terrible. The kids live on hamburgers and Cokes. I'd say you must supplement that diet with something. You can get very good vitamins cheaply at drugstores, get vitamin and mineral supplements, protein supplements, dietary supplements, but the point is you must have something in addition to the food that you are eating normally day by day. It's not really as important for an older fellow as it is for the kids because they are growing organisms, and they really need a good, solid nutritional foundation.

What do you think about nuts, honey, fruits—fresh and dried—and raw sugar?

Great, natural foods are great. Unfortunately, a lot of our kids don't like them. I don't know why not, but I've always been a great lover of nuts and natural foods. It's the best thing we can eat. Let's face it, the human body wasn't designed to be carnivorous. Man can live without meat, but he can't live without natural foods.

Is it your feeling that it would be well to give these to boys in their diet, say, a weekly diet?

We are planning that they have some brown rice and oats so they get all of the cereals during the course of a week's time, not particularly mixed, but so they get grain. As you know, our grain and wheat are from Kansas; our corn from Iowa; oats from somewhere in the north; our rye and rice and barley from various places. Also fruits that are grown in the north, such as apples, or citrus in the south, or the nuts and pecans that are grown in southeastern United States and out on the West Coast—we get so many of our fruits, nuts, almonds, we have a diet scattered rather widely over America, including our cereals and fruits, as well as a good variety of vegetables, especially fresh when they can be had. We showed them what they could expect if they really had an all-year-round training camp.

This was down at York?

This was at York 1960.

How many boys did you have then?

The first year I had 14; the second year I had 17. There were usually 14, 15, or 17 for the next couple of years. But actually I'll tell you something we found out, something very interesting. After two weeks of all this intensive training, where everybody figured these boys would be dead, we staged a little impromptu competition, and the fellows all did much better than they had before in their lives. That's the proof, you know. It proves that the fellows hadn't been working up to standard, working as hard as they could work, but we have a tendency to look at the Bulgarians and Russians and say, well, these fellows have everything their own way, but you've got to remember they are training at least twice or three times as hard as any of our fellows.

That brings in the Bulgarian, the Bulgarian type of training. They train about 5 times a week, don't they? Seven hours a day?

They will train as often as 7 days a week. Normally they train 5 days a week, but then their rest days are active rests; in other words, they are not just lying around on their duff. These fellows are out running, or jumping, or cycling, playing soccer, or swimming, or some other form of pretty good physical activity. It really amounts to a 7-day week.

Now, are they really training 5 hours a day?

Depending upon the season of the year—they train in cycles. During the spring cycle, for example, they will only train about 3 hours a day because during the spring cycle they are handling very heavy poundage and doing a lot of auxiliary exercise. Before competition they lighten the load and train longer so as to get the body up for the stresses they are going to have to endure during competition. So what they do is increase the intensity by having the weights heavy, but by not doing as many repetitions they actually lighten their training load. Their coaches work these things out quite scientifically.

Don't they start boys rather young?

The Bulgarians do, yes, but there again, we do too. We have Junior Olympics 12 years of age.

They start them at 12, is that right?

Just about. Don't forget that a 12-year-old youngster in Bulgaria has already had 5 or 6 years of hard physical training in some other field— light athletics, gymnastics, soccer or something of that nature.

I see. He's been playing since he's been 6 years old.

He's been involved in physical activity for a number of years.

In other words, he's a much more mature all-around athlete at 12 years old than the boy we run into in the first year in high school, who has never done anything.

That's right. When Junius went over to Marseilles, the thing that impressed him the most was the fact that they themselves were 17 years of age, but the Bulgarians they ran across of 17 years were men. They had matured physically because of all the background of training they had. It's a question of maturity through exercise.

What has been the most good weight lifting has done for people?

Well, aside from the competitive angle—winning things, becoming a champion—weight lifting will give a man a degree of self-confidence that he can't get any other way. A fellow who has trained with weights is strong, he's powerful, he hasn't got the sicknesses and little ailments that afflict most everyone else. A weight-trained athlete when he walks down the street tends to swagger and strut, and it's an unconscious thing. He's not trying to show off, but he knows he is good; his body has been developed to the peak of perfection, or he hopes to the peak of perfection. So I think the self-confidence that it imbues in people is probably the greatest thing he can get out of weight lifting.

As to the health aspect, I tell people that I lift weights for insurance. Years of training have made us strong, healthy individuals. I have very little time to train, but the point is physically we have maintained ourselves at a much higher point than the average man simply because we have that background of weight training for years.

We touched on this a little bit ago when you said a boy pushed so hard he injured his hand. What type of injuries have you seen?

Most of the injuries that I've seen have been muscle tears, but lately we're coming up with a new class of injury like the one that_____sustained, the tendons around the knee popping—the patella tendon. I can't really account for something like that. There is something that we are doing wrong that allows the patella tendon to become ruptured.

Well, the first weight lifter I saw—Tommy Kono of Honolulu—was sent by Bob Hoffman and Clarence Johnson. Now they sent these two boys, Charbonneau and McGaule. McGaule is a heavyweight and Charbonneau is a young fellow with a cast on his back. I took them over to Baptist

Hospital where my son, Dick, is in charge of the Physical Therapy Department, and we went over these boys. The main thing that concerns me is of the 40 people we had—weight lifters at Gettysburg, 15 of those people Europeans and Americans—during the period of time that I was with them, which was about 10 days, asked me something about their knees. Now it seems to be under the kneecap down, in the interior part of the kneecap at the tip, right and left of the midline in there.

You're the people that make me immortal in weight training. It's the greatest thing you can get from training with weights. I've seen what happens. You get a youngster who is clearly inhibited and shy and timid, and you can't get him to come out of his shell. He won't talk with people, and he doesn't make friends easily. You bring him into the gymnasium situation and get him trained with weights to the point where his body starts to look like something, and it's the most amazing thing how this fellow's personality will change. He will become more outgoing because he's got a new interest, and he can relate to other people, so I think that would be about the greatest benefit aside from winning championships and things like that, which I don't ever consider that important anymore.

Well, I don't know whether his injury had anything to do with weight lifting because I've seen many discs on many people who never picked up anything heavier than a knife and fork, but Schemansky had two of them, as you know, and each time went back and won medals after each operation. He, of course, was a great specimen, I think we could say one of the great weight lifters of all time.

Without question. When you consider the things that he was doing so many years ago when the rules were so much more stringent than they are now, and the fact that he lasted so many years. I saw the man in competition when he was 46, and he made his best lifetime lift at that point. This is incredible. In any other sport an athlete is washed up. He pulled one of his hamstrings, and he stood a different way to develop the other side of that leg. With a little luck he could have been in the fifth Olympics, and he worked on that really diligently. I think I learned much practical anatomy about the hamstring and quadriceps from Norbert Schemansky, a great student of kinesiology.

Well, he has a lot more muscles to look at. He has massive development, really. With weight lifters who take steroids to gain weight, do you think it's true that the additional weight is held probably by water retention?

A lot of it, an awful lot of it, and some of the throwers seem to think that by adding this weight they lift better. You know, the theory is that by gaining weight like this they are gaining mass, and mass will change the leverages by changing cross-sectional areas of the lift.

Well, the Bulgarians are beginning to make it look that way, don't you think? They look more like athletes.

Yes, indeed, they look very trim.

Now, when some of these men put up a bar, they get under it and put it up, and they are walking around, and the bar is not horizontal, and they can't stabilize that bar. Some of these people have a short leg. Say the short leg is on the right; now the bar is maybe 2 or 3 inches lower down on the right. What do you think when these people are trying to stabilize weight and they can't, so many times they try so long until finally the man tells them to put it down, or they drop it because they can't hold it longer? Why do you think that happens?

Some of it is actually faulty technique. You know, if you practice the proper technique, you can overcome a real physical disability.

We were talking about Schemansky and said he probably was one of the great lifters of all time. In that group, would you classify Tommy Kono and Bob Bednarski?

I would classify Kono, Davis, and Schemansky, but Bednarski, I don't know.

Tommy won the "Mr. Universe," didn't he?

Tommy won "Mr. Universe" and "Mr. World." He was an all-round athlete, really an excellent gymnast, swimmer and diver; an athlete really should excel in not just one sport.

Why do you think the Cubans have come on so fast in the last 6 or 7 years? They've come from nowhere, and all of a sudden they are dominating the American scene.

This is an area in which they felt they could make a lot of progress, and by concentrating on it, they made progress. The Cubans are never going to get anywhere in world basketball. They just don't have that type of person there. Cubans are not naturally big people. Baseball, yes, but baseball is not an Olympic sport. So they had to look around for an Olympic sport that they could shine in. The easiest one to shine in would be weight lifting. It's very simple. They could set up weight-lifting gyms in every little hamlet in the country there, and it's not that big a country. Of course, the weight-lifting equipment is about the easiest thing the government could invest in. The stuff doesn't wear out, it's hard to steal, and it doesn't break.

I never thought about how difficult it would be to steal a set of barbells. What do you think of the training facilities over there?

Oh, they are fantastic. You saw the training halls.

Yes, I thought they were, too.

I thought the hall was the best I'd ever seen. Much better than the Russians', quite frankly, much better. I have never seen the Bulgarian training hall, but I would venture to say they'd be very hard put to exceed the Cubans in that respect.

Our men so many times have to work someplace really like a garage, or someplace they can set up, or get to a Y, as our best facilities are usually in most areas of the country: at least that was true in Detroit. It's true in a lot of areas, unfortunately. There are very few places that are really designed for weight lifting. For example, Y.M.C.A.s are not really designed for weight lifting—mostly for body building and weight training, but not weight lifting. If it wasn't for Clarence Johnson, I don't think we would have had a good weight-lifting room in the Northern Y in Detroit, but that was only on account of Clarence.

I've heard it said many times that weight lifting is the most exact and the fastest of all sports, for you've got to get right in that groove going up; if you're an inch forward or an inch backward, not in a straight line, your drive, your split, or your squat, and your arms under it while you're down, that you slip. Is this true?

To a great extent, it's true. The only thing I would say it's not as exact perhaps as the high dive or gymnastics to some degree, but in weight lifting there's no turning back. I'm against some of these fellows who are so conscious of the exact angle, the back must be at exactly 140° and the spine must be exactly 145°. This is some of the stuff that we've been hearing lately, you know, but it's not true because of the difference in physiological build of one man to another. While my body may function at 140° and the guy I'm coaching is better at 145°, should I impose my thing on him? I can't do it.

Dr. Ono sent me a writing from his university on studies they have done on Berger, Martin, Schemansky, and one other I didn't know, and they showed the line the lift was set on and how the line was when they drove this lift up—it was on the snatch—and how they went up on this and showed the line. Four lines were all different. I noticed Martin's was almost straight. Now you've probably seen those.

Yes, those are the tracings that they made. Again, it's the individual differences in body structure, but sometimes one fellow has a better technique. We know that a straight line is the shortest distance between two points, but you can't pull in a straight line. If you did, you'd bump into your knees when you got the weight off the floor. You must have a slight out curve to get past the knees. Nowadays we pull it into the crotch; in the old days they tried to pull it straight up and down, and now we deliberately pull it in to get our hips under it, and get a lift off the crotch, especially since they've relaxed the rules. Now you can touch the bar with your body and take advantage of everything you can get. You can kick it up with your crotch. So there is a definite wavy line, it's a curve, it's almost like an inverted *S* curve with a hook at the top. The weight will be pulled up past a certain point and then settled down as the lifter drops into his low position. Those are the tracings you are referring to. Every man is different. I don't believe you can follow one pattern.

So many people have asked me if those people are muscle-bound. I have never seen a muscle-bound weight lifter.

As a matter of fact, I invite people to try to do some of the things that I do, not with weights, just bending and twisting and turning and moving the body. A weight lifter can't afford to be muscle-bound because, as I say, if he operates his muscles over a complete range of extension and contraction, the muscles become more flexible. It's only a body builder who might work in half movements to develop a puff; he might end up with an inability to stretch back to a certain point. The body builder's body is so healthy looking to the average person, he thinks, oh, he must be muscle-bound. John Griffith certainly disproved the muscle-bound theory. He performed splits, cupped his hands behind his back in all kinds of movements. The average weight lifter is a pretty flexible guy, he has to be.

What about the fellows you've watched? They start out in weight lifting, go along—what's their success in life compared to a good basketball player? A successful weight lifter has his place. Where does he finish? In the legislature, in a degree of finance how many of them are bums or alcoholics compared with other athletes?

Strangely enough, we have fewer bums. We have a lot of weight lifters who have gone on, you know, fellows like Joe Pittman, who is principal of a high school, Dr. Pete George, who is president of the American Dental Association in Hawaii. We have Vic Kellar, who is an attorney. We have all kinds of people who are successful businessmen, successful people in all walks of life, a lot of schoolteachers and professional people. A tremendous number of weight lifters are schoolteachers, and not just gym teachers—I mean all branches of learning. So I'd say we have a pretty good track record. We may not end up with the financial gains of the football star or the basketball star.

Thank you.

THE BEST MEMORY SYSTEM

Forget each kindness that you do
As soon as you have done it;

Forget the praise that falls on you
The moment you have won it.

Forget the slander that you hear
Before you can repeat it;

Forget each slight, each spite, each sneer,
Wherever you may meet it.

Remember every kindness done
To you, whate'er its measure;

Remember praise by others won
And pass it on with pleasure:

Remember every promise made
And keep it to the letter;

Remember those who lend you aid
And be a grateful debtor.

Remember all the happiness
That comes your way in living;

Forget each worry and distress,
Be hopeful and forgiving;

Remember good, remember truth,
Remember heaven's above you,

And you will find, through age and youth,
That many hearts will love you.

                                   AUTHOR UNKNOWN